Praise for *Walking on Air*

"I think everyone on the face of the E:
In her inspiring book, *Walking on Air*
choices for how to rejuvenate our bodi   ...to toe in just 30
days. With each page of this reader-friendly volume, you will have all
the tools and building blocks you need to create a life of high-level success, health, happiness, and peace."

—**Rafer Johnson,** national head coach, Special Olympics;
Decathlon Olympic Medalist, 1956 Silver, 1960 Gold

"Live this book as Susan lives it and you will have joy dancing in your
heart and the Divine illuminating every thought. *Walking on Air* is an
extraordinary, enlightening book and is a living documentary for creating health and peace with every breath and choice of your life."

—**Gabriel Cousens, MD,** holistic physician and
author of *There Is a Cure for Diabetes*

"The great Peace Corps of planet Earth is its over six billion people.
Anyone who reads Susan's remarkable book, *Walking on Air*, will
become a peacemaker, an instrument of God, and, moreover, will find
health, long life, and happiness."

—**Robert Muller,** former Chancellor of the University
for Peace in Costa Rica and former United Nations
Assistant Secretary-General

"If we lived as Susan suggests, America could close most of its hospitals
and jails and become a nation at peace with itself. She provides an
easy-to-follow 30-day program that is practical, fun, and motivating.
When you finish the 30 days, you will feel and look rejuvenated from
the inside out. I'm going to incorporate this program every month to
help me look and feel my very best throughout the 12 months of the
year. *Walking on Air* is definitely essential reading for everyone."

—**Nick Lawrence,** *BBC Radio 4* talk-show host

"*Walking on Air* is a book all of us need to read not just once, but over and over again. Susan takes the reader on a journey within, where we find the happiness, balance, rejuvenation, and peace to become the living person we truly are."

—**Barbara De Angelis, PhD,**
author of *How Did I Get Here?*

"Susan's writing and presence continually inspire and remind me that health, inner peace, and a joyful heart are available to me if I choose them. She is a master teacher of a balanced path of strength and heart. If you follow her guidance in *Walking on Air*, you will be able to create the body of your dreams and the best health of your life. Everyone should read this life-changing work. I love all of her books, but this one may very well be my favorite. Kudos to Susan!"

—**Alan Cohen,** author of *A Daily Dose of Sanity*

"If you would like some practical, effective ways to deal with stress; if you desire to be healthier, happier, or more peaceful; if you want some insightful guidance on how to live a more balanced life; or if you simply want to enrich your experience of living, making your life a great adventure and reveling in life's simple pleasures, then *Walking on Air* is perfect for you. Susan will empower and motivate you to let go of your excuses, to move in the direction of your dreams, and to create your very best life—and in record-breaking time, too."

—**Victoria Moran,** author of *Creating a Charmed Life*

"An outstanding guide to rejuvenating your body, mind, and spirit and living a life that is rooted in the eternal source."

—**John Robbins,** author of *The Food Revolution*

"Books that I love become more than ink on paper; they become good friends. Long after they are read, even sitting on the shelf, their vibrations continue to bless, heal, enrich, and nurture me. Susan's powerful and life-transforming book *Walking on Air* is destined to be such a friend."

—**Rev. John Strickland,** Unity minister

"Susan offers us a life-changing, 30-day healthy living makeover program in *Walking on Air*. She provides us with the information and guidance that we can all incorporate for increased prosperity, whole-body rejuvenation, personal peace, and longevity for ourselves and our planet Earth."

—**Elson M. Haas, MD,** author of *More Vegetables, Please!*

"Susan's enthusiasm, experience, and vast knowledge of the current fields of optimal nutrition, exercise, human potential, and wellness are great gifts. I saw her speak recently to an audience of about a thousand, and it was as if an angel of joy and wisdom had been dropped into our midst. If you are not fortunate enough to attend one of her presentations, then the next best thing is to read this book and apply its down-to-earth tips, which you'll find on every page."

—**Anita Finley,** *Anita Finley Radio Talk Show* host and
publisher of *Boomer Times*

"When you discover a way to profoundly change your life, you never look back. Invite Susan Smith Jones to guide you to vibrant health and youthful vitality."

—**Neal Barnard, MD**

"As you apply Susan's suggestions in your kitchen and life, you'll be embarking on a great adventure in both self-care and compassion."

—**Victoria Moran**

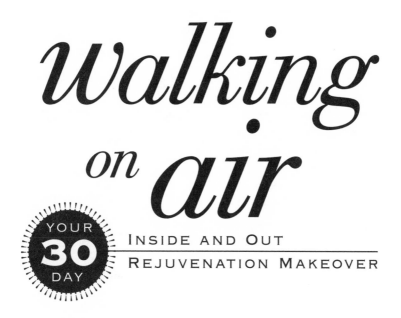

Walking on air

YOUR **30** DAY

INSIDE AND OUT
REJUVENATION MAKEOVER

SUSAN SMITH JONES, PhD

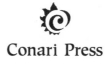

Conari Press

First published in 2011
by Conari Press, an imprint of
Red Wheel/Weiser, LLC
With offices at:
665 Third Street, Suite 400
San Francisco, CA 94107
www.redwheelweiser.com

ISBN: 978-1-57324-497-8

Library of Congress Cataloging-in-Publication Data

Jones, Susan Smith, 1950-
   Walking on air : your 30-day inside and out rejuvenation makeover / Susan
Smith Jones.
      p.   cm.
   ISBN 978-1-57324-497-8 (alk. paper)
   1. Self-care, Health. I. Title.
   RA776.95.J66 2011
   613—dc22

                                                          2011007029

Cover design by Barb Fisher
Text design by ContentWorks, Inc.
Cover photograph © Edmund Nagele PCL / SuperStock
Printed in Canada
TCP
10 9 8 7 6 5 4 3 2 1

I joyfully and lovingly dedicate this book to my earth angel, Caroline Pincus—this book's midwife. She took my rejuvenation program and my vision for the book and put wings under it, guiding me every step of the way. Without her caring, warmhearted, and gracious support, this book would not have been written. My deep gratitude and appreciation goes to this beautiful and brilliant soul, whom I'm so proud to call my dear friend.

This book is also dedicated to my Aunt Jackie, who inspires me with her independent, generous spirit and passion for life. She has a heart of gold and is always showing me, by example, the importance of living by the golden rule.

Contents

Foreword

by Alexandra Stoddard

In our being we hold the ability to have vibrant physical health and to create a gracious life intentionally filled with blessings. This book offers us the keys to achieving these goals through daily affirmations and positive action steps that will bring us closer to the ideal life we've always dreamed of having.

Walking on Air can mean so many things—floating along on a transparently golden summer day, an inner lightness that buoys us up through any mood, or a sense of being lifted along by a Higher Power. In this instructive manual written from the heart and including scientific research, Susan Smith Jones, PhD, shows readers how to achieve this enlightened state by attending to the trinity of mind, body, and spirit. The result gives us an indescribable feeling of buoyant inner power.

Most of us want to improve our lives continuously—simply living, trying to find our own path on a quest to live a more effective and enjoyable life as we seek deeper answers to the problems we encounter and question large philosophical issues we wish to understand better. By drawing from the great minds of history, as well as a range of literary, spiritual, and contemporary sources, Susan presents the reader with nuggets of wisdom to savor, first by opening every chapter with an intriguing quotation, and then by closing with another thoughtful insight.

Walking on Air isn't just meant to feed the mind—it's a plan for daily action, created to leave you, thirty days later, in a healthier, more vibrant state of mind, body, and soul. By considering the food you eat, taking time to be alone, and assessing your higher consciousness, while simplifying your life and returning to a connection with nature, you will feel stronger, more relaxed, and eager to take on the challenges in your life.

Busy lives inevitably create a hectic pace of life and, unfortunately, experiencing beauty, feeling wonder, and breathing deeply of nature's blessings often fall to the bottom of our to-do lists. Susan's inspiring book will help us reconsider our priorities and reassess how we use our time and what we value in order to live a more fully realized life. The secret to creating these transforming changes is that they're made daily, incrementally, and they build on one another, so that nothing becomes a burden, but rather, the cumulative effect of manageable steps carries us forward.

It's not easy to start a new life-changing program or to give up old habits. Fortunately, *Walking on Air* is a nurturing guide. Listening to Susan's advice and, consequently, to that of her grandmother (Fritzie) and her mother (June) reminds us of listening to an old friend reaching across the kitchen table to share both common sense and uncommon wisdom. This book is practical to read and delightfully pleasant to follow. If we commit ourselves to this thirty-day plan and its daily principles, we'll find that in just one month's time, we'll feel stronger, happier, healthier, and more serene, restored, and ready to soar.

—**Alexandra Stoddard**, author of *You Are Your Choices*, *Things I Want My Daughters to Know*, *Things Good Mothers Know*, *Living a Beautiful Life*, *Happiness for Two*, and many others
www.AlexandraStoddard.com

Author's Note

The health suggestions and recommendations in this book are based on the training, research, and personal experiences of the author. Because each person and situation is unique, the author and publisher encourage the reader to check with his or her holistic physician or other health professional before using any procedure outlined in this book. It is a sign of wisdom to seek a second or third opinion. Neither the author nor the publisher is responsible for any adverse consequences resulting from a change in diet or from the use of any other suggestions in this book.

Introduction

There is a blessing in the air.

—William Wordsworth

Do not go where the path may lead.
Go instead where there is no path and leave a trail.

—Ralph Waldo Emerson

If you've picked up this book, chances are that you are seeking change in your life—not just a new hairstyle or a fresh wardrobe, but lasting, meaningful, and resounding change for your sense of health and happiness.

You have definitely come to the right place! *Walking on Air* is a compendium of wisdom that reveals how to create a life of robust self-esteem, vibrant physical health, and deepened spiritual consciousness. The wisdom in the book is culled from over thirty-five years of experience as an educator, consultant, and motivational speaker in the fields of holistic health and human potential. But I haven't just studied how to make lasting change in your life—I've lived it! And, for me, the catalysts of change have often arrived in packages I was not expecting.

We've all heard the clichés "Change begins with you" or "Change begins with choice." Though it's true that authentic transformation comes from within and modifying your life necessitates a deliberate commitment to new thoughts and behaviors, sometimes the catalysts of change are delivered from external sources. That has definitely been the case in my life. As you embark on your journey of change, using this book as your companion, I'd like to first share some of my life-altering experiences to offer hope and guidance to light your path.

The Mind-Body-Spirit Connection

When I was seventeen, my father unexpectedly passed away. I was devastated. I had no precedent for this type of deep loss and no skills to cope with it. My way of dealing with the tragedy was, really, by not dealing with it at all. I stuffed all my feelings inside and numbed myself with food—typical teenage temptations of fast-food burgers, pizza, and sugary sweets and pastries galore. Today I would recognize this bingeing behavior as a hallmark of depression, but back then I didn't realize what was going on. After a year of managing my grief by eating everything in sight, my health took a nosedive. I developed allergies, asthma, acne, and arthritis, not to mention I had gained a considerable amount of weight.

While I suffered physically, the emotional toll was even greater. Before my father's death, I had been an active and social teenager. Now an overweight high school student with acne, I became the subject of jokes around campus and was bullied by people I'd thought were my friends. I was rapidly losing any semblance of confidence and self-esteem. My heart was heavy, and I was sinking emotionally. Pain was devouring my will to live. It was not a pretty picture.

Luckily for me, there was another catalyst of change already present in my life: my beloved grandmother, whom I called Fritzie. Like many grandmothers, Fritzie was kind, nurturing, and full of wisdom, but she also possessed a vast wealth of knowledge about health and the human body. When she saw my physical and emotional state a year after my father's passing, she knew immediately that I needed healing from the inside out.

Her first step was to take me to our family doctor for a checkup to make sure no life-threatening disease had taken hold. When I told the doctor my symptoms, he apprised me that I would have to live with my newly developed allergies, asthma, arthritis, and acne the rest of my life because, as he said, it was in my genes. Leaving his office with a handful of prescriptions that he implored us to fill immediately, I felt even more depressed and powerless.

My grandmother, in all her wisdom, instead took me home and had a heart-to-heart talk with me. She told me that if I followed her suggestions 100 percent, my health issues and depression would disappear within thirty days. She said my acne would clear up, my asthma would dissipate, my energy would soar, my extra weight would melt away, and my attitude would change from negative and powerless to positive and hopeful.

Needless to say, she had my attention. A wise person once said, "When the student is ready, the teacher will appear," and this was definitely true for me. I was ready.

Fritzie started by overhauling my diet of snack foods and sweets. She was an advocate of eating foods as close to the way nature made them as possible. "In nature," she firmly reminded me, "we won't find ice cream trees, potato chip bushes, or doughnut vines." Though I initially resisted eating the colorful vegetables, fresh juices, sprouts, and other living foods that she prepared for me (what teenager wouldn't?), soon enough I became a believer. The pounds started coming off, my skin became clear and vibrant again, my asthma was soothed, and my outlook improved.

Fritzie also went to work on healing my spirit. She knew that the underlying cause of my poor diet and physical ailments was the loss of my father. I would often hear her say, "The body reflects the mind, and the mind reflects the spirit." She explained to me that even when our lives are burdened with loss and tragedy, we can still find much to be grateful for. The first thing she taught me was to begin each day blessing everything—the sunrise, the sound of the mourning doves, my unlimited opportunities, my potential to create whatever I wanted, and anything I had planned for the day.

Fritzie helped me cultivate and choose an attitude of gratitude, which included speaking only positive words and affirmations, even when appearances showed me the opposite. Her voice is ingrained in my mind saying, "Attitude is the mind's paintbrush; it can color anything." She suggested that I recite these two affirmations daily: "I behold the divine in everyone and everything," and "Only the best for me." I was surprised by how approaching each day from a perspective of hope and gratitude began to assuage my grief for my father. I started to see the world once again as an inviting, abundant place.

At the end of the thirty days, astounding transformations had occurred. Not only had I seen dramatic improvements in my health, appearance, and attitude, but the tools for lasting change had taken root. With all Fritzie's wisdom and down-to-earth common sense, she had enlightened me on the benefits of taking care of my body from head to toe, inside and out. I learned to listen to my body's whisperings and to look to God's bounty of natural remedies. It felt like a new and glorious way to live—in God's hands with nature's treasure trove as my partner. I threw the doctor's prescriptions away.

In this book, I hope to be a catalyst of change for you, just as Fritzie was for me. Though the wealth of information in *Walking on Air* has been selected from many years of study and my experience working with thousands of people around the world, Fritzie's common-sense teachings are its foundations. Ultimately, change must come from inside, but that doesn't mean you don't need the loving hand of a knowledgeable guide to start you down the path.

A Leap of Faith

In the years after I recovered from grieving for my father, I felt as if I could conquer any problem that came my way and that my vibrant health was foolproof. I kept a diet loaded with fresh fruits and vegetables, an active lifestyle (I loved baseball and once dreamed of being the first female L.A. Dodgers player!), and an outlook of gratitude and positivity. As long as I continued to tend to my mind, body, and spirit, I felt I was invincible.

But of course, the Universe is never static, and change came knocking on my door once again. In my twenties, I was in a terrible automobile accident. Though I felt lucky to have survived, I fractured my back so badly that doctors told me I would never again be physically active and would have chronic pain the rest of my life. I plunged into despair because all of a sudden my life and my body no longer felt like they were in my control.

Though Fritzie's tactics had helped me shed pounds and regain balance as a teenager, I knew they wouldn't be enough to heal a fractured back. One evening while sitting in silence on a bench at sunset, gazing at the ocean near my home in west Los Angeles and searching for answers, I had a sudden epiphany. I felt God's loving presence, and I knew that His plan for me wasn't a life of pain. All at once, I realized the tool I had been missing was *faith*. In all his sagacity, Ralph Waldo Emerson wrote this soul-stirring sentence: "The whole course of things goes to teach us faith." I love this passage and remind myself of its profundity every day, especially when life sends me a curveball.

In an instant, I rejected the doctor's prognosis and resolved to prove him wrong. From that day forward, I decided to live only from a place of optimism. Although the next few months were filled with pain, I endured. I attended lectures and read numerous books on the power of commitment in physical healing, and I never let my faith in my ability to heal waver.

When I visited my doctor for a follow-up appointment six months later, he shook his head in bewilderment. "This just can't be," he said. "There is no sign of a fracture, and you seem to be in perfect health, free of pain. There must be some mistake. It's just miraculous." Through my determination, along with the mind-body-spirit practices I'd learned from Fritzie, my back had managed to heal completely! Far from living a life of disability and chronic pain, I resumed fitness activities, and today I regularly participate in hiking, weight training, inline skating, biking, horseback riding, Pilates, and yoga.

I now see that accident as the impetus to changing my life for the better. My recovery proved that we have within ourselves everything we need to live life to the fullest. But we also need to learn from others who've walked the path we want to walk. I credit the individuals who shared their experiences through lectures, books, and conversations during that painful time as endowing me with the tools I needed to spearhead my own recovery.

Now, years later, I am at the other end of the spectrum, as my teachings, books, and life principles help others to live joyful, soul-satisfying lives. Gratefully, I now have an enthusiastic following and am in demand internationally as a health and fitness expert, personal growth specialist, leadership consultant, retreat leader, and motivational speaker for corporate, community, church, spiritual, and women's groups. I strive to spread the message that *anyone* can choose radiant health and physical, mental, and spiritual rejuvenation. That's why I've written *Walking on Air,* so that you, too, can shape your own healing and live to your highest potential.

The sunflower has always been one of my favorite flowers. I love how its wide face is so open, how its yellow leaves brighten any room, and how, as a heliotrope, it naturally seeks the sun. I also love eating raw sunflower seeds and making sunflower seed milk and cheese (nondairy), and I enjoy any salad, smoothie, or other dish that includes sunflower green sprouts as well. When I was a child, I used to make up songs about sunflowers, as they seemed like a natural companion to my own optimistic nature.

As an avid gardener, horticulturist, and enthusiast on anything related to flowers, plants, and gardening, I was reminded of this flower connection recently, as I listened to a news report on the radio about daffodils. I heard this remarkable comment from a scientist being interviewed. He said, "Humans share 35 percent of their DNA with daffodils." Does that surprise you, too? That flower-human connection made me think more about sunflowers. I remember how much I felt the sunflower was almost an alter ego to myself and how fundamental our connection is to the natural world. Just as the sunflower turns its face toward the sun to grow and to thrive, we must also face the outer light while tending to our own budding seeds. We each blossom when planted in fertile soil and nourished with food and care. We can be the caretakers of our own growth, just as we tend to our plants, pets, and loved ones. Now is the time to let your newly nurtured roots gather strength in order to bloom.

How to Use This Book

As a holistic lifestyle coach, I work with only a few select clients each year so that I can offer my utmost energy and vitality to each. Previous clients have included corporate presidents, politicians, world-class athletes, and everyday people who want to achieve a greater sense of purpose. Working on all levels—physical, mental, emotional, and spiritual—I teach my clients how to incorporate my gold-star secrets to being vibrantly healthy and stunningly successful. With a copy of *Walking on Air* in hand, think of yourself as one of my personal clients— you now have at your fingertips all of my tools and advice to take your life from ordinary to extraordinary! Just for you, I have put decades of invaluable information and research into this reader-friendly book. I imagine you sitting across from me at my kitchen table right now as we begin a friendly chat, one in which I wish to convey how much I want the best health possible for you, as well as inner peace. I hope you will understand how dearly I value these principles for myself and want to extend their benefits to everyone I know and care about—and that includes you.

If you have already peeked at the table of contents, you will see a theme involving three of my favorite words: *Choose, Cultivate,* and *Celebrate*. For me, this is what we all need every day—to choose the best, to cultivate a holistic lifestyle, and to celebrate our blessings.

Our countless daily choices determine our level of health and how we feel. And there are three choices over which we always have control: what we eat, how we move (exercise), and what we think. And we have the power to change these at any time. We also have the power to cultivate our dreams and to celebrate each day. The power of choice is what living fully and successfully is all about.

The saying "The ancients have stolen all our best ideas" remains true. What I'm writing about isn't new, but it's fresh in that it's written from my perspective (combined with the wisdom of my grandmother and my mother) and daily experiences. For example, I meditate every day, but on a few special days during the week, I couple this ritual with a sunrise hike. I am able to do this year-round because I have the privilege of living in sunny Los Angeles, my hometown. This is my time, when I let nature lift my spirit and nurture my soul. As you'll see in this book, my sunrise hikes allow me to practice the principles "Celebrate Salubrious Silence and Solitude" and "Celebrate the Miracle of Your Body with Exercise."

I also regularly practice the principle "Choose to Lighten Up and Be Childlike." I simply love to laugh (I'm known to be a practical joker)! My mother, June, called laughter "the body's elixir" or natural rejuvenator. It is an essential ingredient to daily living and something I use to fuel my spirituality. Because of my positive, easygoing, lighten-up approach to life, I have acquired the nickname "Sunny" because I am always reminding others not to take life so seriously.

Another theme central to my daily experience is boosting my self-esteem. No matter where I travel and with whom I work, I believe the thing people wrestle with most in their own lives is loss of faith in themselves, in other words, low self-esteem. In my own life, I fortify self-esteem through the principles "Choose to Be CEO of Your Body and Life" and "Cultivate the Art of Perseverance and Determination," among others. If we remain in control of our own lives, meet our goals day by day, and treat ourselves with tenderness, our self-esteem will blossom.

These are just a few of the thirty principles I rely upon in my own life and in my practice as a holistic lifestyle coach, and they are all my gifts to you in *Walking on Air*. You may not agree with my chosen path or what I write; all I ask is that you keep your heart tender and your mind open.

I suggest that you read this book through once in its entirety. Then read it again, slowly and deliberately, reading no more than one chapter a day for 30 days. This is a 30-day, inside and out, rejuvenation program for your body, mind, and spirit. I've chosen this time frame because it is doable, and—believe me—it is enough time for you to see significant differences in how you look and feel. Think about the topic for the day. Absorb it. Practice living it, and make sure you participate in "Today's Affirmation & Action Step" at the end of each chapter. Each step builds on the day before, and by the end of the book, you will be well on your way to a renewed and enriched life and to feeling like you are walking on air.

Books are more than just words on a page. You, the reader, bring the words to life. Apply what you read, and look for ways you can experience more celebration in your life than you've ever felt before. I love what Henry David Thoreau said about the books he preferred to read:

> Books, not which afford us a cowering enjoyment,
> but in which each thought is of unusual daring; such
> as an idle person cannot read, and a timid one would
> not be entertained by, which even make us dangerous
> to existing institutions—such I call good books.

My hope is that this book cultivates the same sense of "unusual daring" in you to take charge of your life in a powerful way. If you feel stuck, like you're in a spin-cycle lifestyle, if you've lost some of your joy and would like to experience more lasting happiness, or if you just need some gentle, loving, efficacious guidance to live in a more meaningful way, you will find here the catalyst you need.

There is no time like the present. Make your life the magnificent adventure it was created to be. I salute your great adventure, and I wish you the daily feeling that you are walking on air.

～

Two roads diverged in a wood, and I—I took the one least traveled by, and that has made all the difference.

—Robert Frost

"Be quick but don't hurry." By that, I meant make a decision, take action; decide what you're going to do and do it. Keep this word of caution in mind: Failure to act is often the biggest failure of all.

—Coach John Wooden

Walking on Air

Day 1

Celebrate Yourself and Live Fully

The meaning of things lies not in the things themselves but in our attitude toward them.

—ANTOINE DE SAINT-EXUPÉRY

You cannot make yourself feel something you do not feel, but you can make yourself do right in spite of your feelings.

—PEARL S. BUCK

Think about this: eighty billion humans have walked this planet since the beginning of time, and never has there been anyone exactly like you. If each of the almost seven billion people living on our planet right now were to stream by you in single file, it would take two hundred years to greet each one in turn. How miraculous is that? In two hundred years you would never find two people exactly alike. You would never find two whose experiences had been the same or whose fingerprints were alike or who thought, believed, felt, or talked alike.

To that, let's add another amazing fact. Of the approximately fifty million to a hundred million sperm that traveled an immense distance, overcame tremendous obstacles, just one won the competition— probably the fiercest and most challenging of its life—and succeeded at fertilizing the one egg that lay in wait and together they joined to become you. You see, you are already a winner.

What's more, you are composed of a body, mind, and spirit, and you already have everything you need to live up to your highest potential—to become master of your life. I think that calls for a celebration.

Today, as we begin our 30 days together, I ask you to focus on this miracle, this work of divinity that is you. The world-respected spiritual teacher Paramahansa Yogananda used to tell his students, "A little gram of your flesh contains enough latent energy to keep the city of Chicago supplied with electricity for a week. And yet," he continued, "you complain of feeling tired! It is because you live too much attached to the body, rather than seeing yourselves as waves of God's infinite energy!"

If the word God does not feel comfortable to you, please replace it with something else, such as Love, Light, Inner Light, Infinite Joy, Creator, Higher Power, Loving Presence, God-Light, Love-Light, Divine Mind, Divine Power, Angels, All-Peace, Lord, the Divine, Heart-Light, Spirit, or anything else that feels best for you. I'll use different references for the word God from time to time throughout this book. The point is, we are all waves of divine and infinite energy and potential, and I encourage you to spend some time thinking about that today.

It's so easy to identify with the way our bodies look. Just last week I saw a television program about plastic surgery in which they interviewed teenagers who were unhappy with their looks. They were getting all types of plastic surgery—breast implants, having ribs removed to make their waists smaller, cheek and chin implants, liposuction, and lip injections. It was heartbreaking to see teenagers so determined to change their bodies to suit some cultural ideal and worse yet that their parents were supporting them in creating the "bodies of their dreams." It was fairly obvious that the parents didn't feel good about their own bodies and were passing that judging attitude on to their children.

Of course, we are all encouraged to improve our appearances all the time. Just look at most magazine ads or television commercials. Either by innuendo or by outright declaration, they encourage us to change who we are in some fundamental way. Here's the truth of the matter: you can spend millions of dollars changing your physical features, but that will do little good until you stop looking for love and acceptance from the outside in.

When you are not feeling good about you, you feel separated from others and God. When you see yourself as a failure, you create a self-fulfilling prophecy. You attract to yourself that which you believe you deserve. Your negative thoughts and attitudes about yourself, whether they originated within yourself or others, convince you of your inability to succeed. If you feel you don't deserve success, prosperity, happy relationships, joy, and peace, then you're settling for less than you are entitled. When you feel unworthy, you cut yourself off from the fullness of life.

Unconditional self-love and self-acceptance can disconnect this vicious cycle. Through inner work, we can develop genuine self-esteem, self-confidence, self-respect, and self-appreciation. We must go beyond our limiting beliefs and realize our importance to ourselves and to the world. Each of us is unique and has something very special to offer. Our Creator doesn't make any mistakes. Understand that you have always done your best at any given time; you don't have to be so hard on yourself. And now, you have the opportunity to choose again.

At any moment, we have a choice: to judge ourselves, or to be kind and loving. Whether we succeed or fail, enjoy our lives or struggle, depends largely on how we view ourselves. In fact, numerous studies have concluded that the key to taking control of our lives is changing the view we have of ourselves.

Loving ourselves, feeling good about ourselves, is an inside job. When you begin to see yourself as divine, chances are you'll be happy with the miraculous physical body that your Creator provided for you, and you will establish a salutary health and fitness program to keep your body temple in peak functioning order.

Today I want you to begin developing a loving relationship with yourself. Think about what it would mean to be your own best friend. Choose to take wonderful care of yourself, your body temple, and your magnificent world. Look within for guidance and the answers to your questions. If you are willing and open, you will find what you have been seeking.

So today, Day 1 of our 30-day program, begin discovering yourself and all the beauty, splendor, and wonder housed within you. You are the only person you can ever know intimately. You are the one with whom you must live eternally. Imagine living as though you are the most special person on planet earth, because you really are.

Who you truly are, deep in your heart, is so much greater than anything you'll ever achieve in life. As Anwar Sadat, former president of Egypt, said, "I have realized that my real self is a greater entity than any possible post or title." Your real self—divine self—is a deep river that connects with God and with all life. At this moment, your real self may be hidden or unexpressed, but it is always available to you, with all its profundity, joy, and wisdom. When attuned to this inner self, we are, in the words of Joseph Campbell, "following our bliss."

When you are living fully, each day brings reason to celebrate, and work and play become one. When you celebrate yourself and life, you find yourself doing what you love to do. Strength, confidence, joy, and peace are the basis of all your experiences. Of course, you will encounter some pain and challenges along the way—this is an inevitable part of being human. But when you are living fully, hardships are short-lived, and you can learn from them and grow and change. Walt Whitman describes splendidly this state of celebrating yourself and life.

> A man realizes the venerable myth—he is a god
> walking the earth, he sees new eligibilities, powers,
> and beauties everywhere; he himself has a new
> eyesight and hearing. The play of the body in
> motion takes a previously unknown grace. Merely
> to move is then a happiness, a pleasure—to breathe,
> to see, is also. All the beforehand gratifications,
> drink, spirits, coffee, grease, stimulants, mixtures,
> late hours, luxuries, deeds of the night, seem as
> vexatious dreams, and now the awakening.

Remember this: your radiant body responds to the blessings of love, praise, and gratitude. Take time each day to bless your body temple and acknowledge your oneness with spirit. Place all your cares, worries, and problems into the Light and ask that only those things necessary for your highest good be returned for your attention.

Celebrate your magnificence.

Do what you can, with what you have, where you are.

—Theodore Roosevelt

Creating is easy if you view the world as if you were a child. Playing and creating are almost synonymous.

—Bernie Siegel

Today's Affirmation & Action Step

The holy presence of Love within me heals my mind and body. I am vitally alive, enthusiastic about my life, and living life to the hilt. Every day is a new adventure of wonder, joy, magnificence, happiness, and peace. I celebrate myself and life.

Do something special today to honor your body temple. Some examples might be to take a bubble bath; splurge on new, luxurious bedding; buy new PJs that feel good against your skin; get a massage, facial, or manicure and pedicure; or anything else that honors and loves your beautiful body temple. Today, think about how miraculous your body is.

Day 2

Choose Uplifting Words, Thoughts, and Imagination

Wisdom is avoiding all thoughts that weaken you.

—Louise L. Hay

Happiness depends more on the inward disposition of mind than on the outward circumstances.

—Benjamin Franklin

Control of the mind is essential if we are going to experience the joy of walking on air. Be firm but loving, for the mind is the reins that control the horses—the emotions and the body—and guides them along the road of life. Train the mind always to see the best in others and in everything. When the road of life is steep, keep your mind even.

Whatever you give your love, time, and attention to will return to you. From within the silence of your being emanates the ability to think, create, and become whatever you want to become. Think only about those things you want to invite into your life. The following quote comes from one of my favorite spiritual books *The Quiet Mind: Sayings of White Eagle*.

In your search for truth, you must continually project thoughts of goodwill and love. Always

see good, even if the good appears infinitesimal
in comparison with other things. Let your
thoughts of love and goodwill be broadcast.

Our lives reflect our thoughts, dreams, expectations, beliefs, hopes, feelings of self-worth, and desires. Knowing this, you can consciously modify your inner state to create a life that reflects your highest potential and vision. We are not victims of circumstance; we are the architects of our lives. We create our own heaven or hell. Complications, conditions, or people should not upset you; rather, the way you think about them will cause your upset.

When we take charge of ourselves, our thoughts, our emotions, our words, and our actions, all things respond. Through the activity of dwelling in heart-light, we have the power to retrain our minds. No matter how long or how often we have misused our minds, we can still mold our thoughts and use them in ways that are positive and uplifting from here on out.

You say you're justified in certain mental patterns because of what's happened in your life? You must break the cycle if you are to create a positive, peaceful, and happy future. As you think, you feel; and as you feel, you radiate; and as you radiate, you attract back the essence of what you express and project. Believe me, it took a few years and loads of discipline to retrain my mind. Until that time, I kept repeating negative patterns in my life. Now I strive to focus my thoughts on what I want for myself and for my world. In so doing, I feel empowered and uplifted. I radiate positive energy, which gives me the magnetic power to attract that which I consider to be salutary. Never underestimate the power of your mind as master controller. Jesus said, "As you think, so shall you be" (Proverbs 23:7). There's no denying that the quality of your thoughts determines the quality of your life.

Albert Einstein wrote, "Imagination is more important than knowledge. For knowledge is limited, whereas imagination embraces the entire world, stimulating progress, giving birth to evolution." He also opined: "Your imagination is a preview of your life's coming attractions." I love that thought! And Émile Coué observed, "When the imagination and the will are in conflict, the imagination invariably gains the day." So, no matter how much we may will something, if we consistently harbor mental pictures that undermine that desire, we won't receive what we will. Coué built a whole therapeutic practice based on the simple affirmation: "Day by day, in every way, I'm getting better and better."

At least once a day, I incorporate conscientious creative visualization into my schedule. Creative visualization is a tool for using your imagination more consciously. You must practice it with thanksgiving and acceptance. If you want greater health, see yourself in your mind's eye as radiantly healthy and energetic. Make these images vivid and real. If you want more peace, visualize yourself as a peaceful person. The same goes for prosperity, creativity, happiness, relationships, or anything else you might want. Imagine your ideal vision and feel the joy and gratitude you would have were the vision your reality. Creative visualization should allow no limits on your thinking and feeling. Stay open to your possibilities.

Use affirmations in conjunction with creative visualization. Be sure to keep your words sweet in case you have to eat them, as the folk wisdom admonishes. Words have power. Speak only words that are loving, true, kind, and helpful. Always speak from your highest self and let your words express the truth of your being. As Jesus said, it is "not what enters his mouth that defiles a man, but what comes out of his mouth" (Matt. 15:11).

Affirmations are an opportunity to speak the truth about who you are and what you want to create. Soon, you'll be doing more than just saying the right words, thinking the right thoughts, and visualizing your goals and dreams. Soon, you will have adopted a whole new way of being, one that aligns what you think with what you feel, and what you say with what you do.

My books *The Joy Factor* and *Healthy, Happy & Radiant . . . at Any Age*, my audiobook *Wired to Meditate*, and my audio program *Celebrate Life!* are all good resources for visualizations and affirmations. These days, most of my visualizations and affirmations have to do with being in perfect harmony with the loving light I see within. I want to be an open vessel through which God's will can manifest in my life. My human mind is not usually aware of what this will for me is, but my Divine Mind knows. Every day, through prayer and meditation, I consciously surrender strength to the radiant power and light within me, holding nothing back; I ask for awareness, strength, and courage to act on the guidance I receive. In adopting this way of living, I have seen more change and had far greater fulfillment in my life than I ever imagined possible. I realize that Spirit can do for me only what it can do through me.

In addition to doing your creative visualization and affirmations, allow yourself time to find out what God's will is for you. Be open. Let peace be your compass on the path to fulfillment and walking on air. Use each Affirmation & Action Step with focus, concentration, and feeling.

Choose uplifting words, thoughts, and imagination today.

~

If you love everything, you will perceive the divine mystery of things.

—FYODOR DOSTOEVSKY

Dare to live the life you have dreamed for yourself. Go forward and make your dreams come true.

—RALPH WALDO EMERSON

Today's Affirmation & Action Step

My peaceful, happy thoughts reflect the Light and Love within me. I focus on what I desire and deserve, for I know that new thoughts create new conditions. I allow Love's thoughts to be my thoughts. I am renewed, regenerated, and restored, for I am living a joyful, healthy life.

If you were living the life of your dreams right now, what would it look like? If you knew you couldn't fail, how would you be living? Write down your response as though this vision were your current reality. Read it often, and feel the joy you would experience in living this life. Return to this vision-reality often during the 30-day program to fertilize the dream. Trust and believe. Think about what you want in your life today.

Day 3

Cultivate a Healthy, Cleansed, and Detoxified Body

Until he extends his circle of compassion to all living things, man will not himself find peace.

—ALBERT SCHWEITZER

The human body is its own best apothecary. The most successful prescriptions are those filled by the body itself.

—NORMAN COUSINS

For centuries, throughout ancient medical traditions the world over, healing practitioners have known the importance of detoxification—drawing out, neutralizing, and eliminating accumulated toxins—for maintaining optimum health. In Ayurvedic practice in India, for example, the definition of health is a state in which the body is free of toxins, organs are functioning optimally, and waste is eliminated efficiently. Similarly, in Chinese medicine, the body's ability to detoxify—to expunge both toxic wastes and negative emotions—is considered the root of both physical and mental well-being. Teas and tonics are among the natural remedies used by Chinese practitioners to rid the body of by-products that accumulate simply from the normal, everyday activities of eating, breathing, and exercising. Native Americans and other indigenous cultures have long used fasting and sweat lodges to purify the body in a comparable way.

Today, we have even more need for detoxification than our ancient forebears. Under ideal conditions, the body's expertly designed detox system expels toxins efficiently. But in modern life, we've come to overtax our systems a great deal. Due to the stresses of our fast-paced society, we are often sleep-deprived, fraught with anxiety, and overfull of nutritionally void fast foods, so our bodies are unable to perform the deeper level of detoxification that is necessary to avert the accumulation of ordinary toxins. Add to this the toxins we've introduced to our world within the past fifty years—synthetic chemicals, air and water pollutants, heavy metals, prescription drugs, and trans-fat acids—and it's clear that we're piling on much more than our natural detoxification systems were designed to handle.

Modern practitioners have begun to investigate the efficacy of ancient healing practices to bolster the body's detox mechanisms. Though many people remain skeptical of detoxification programs (such as intensive juicing and fad fasting cleansing programs) because of the potential health risks they pose, there is a growing consensus that when used properly, herbs and nutritionally rich foods can help coax the body into a deeper level of detox than its normal baseline and thereby quell many conditions associated with toxicity.

Completing a detox program is like working with a clean slate: not only will you help prevent the onset of disease in the long term, you will also notice short-term benefits such as weight loss, clear skin, and renewed energy.

We'd like to think that toxic wastes are only the creation of modern science, but the truth is that our bodies manufacture wastes that are toxic and must constantly engage in toxic waste cleanup. Like a nuclear power plant, each of our trillions of cells is in the business of manufacturing energy. These mini factories are powered by nutrients from the food we eat and oxygen from the air we breathe. As a result of normal metabolism, our cells generate wastes known as endotoxins, which include carbon dioxide, uric acid, ammonia, lactic acid, and homocysteine.

Luckily, our bodies were designed to do their own endotoxin cleanup. Under normal conditions, the waste is released into the circulatory system, neutralized in the blood, and safely passed out of the body via the skin (as sweat), the lungs (as carbon dioxide), the kidneys (as urine), and the intestines (as fecal matter). This process is continuous—it's happening right now as you are sitting and reading and breathing.

Creating energy is what drives our existence, but expunging our waste products is just as crucial to sustaining life. If anything goes wrong with our detoxification systems along the way, toxins build up and can cause disease and death. You may be wondering, if our bodies already take care of their own detoxification, what is the point of engaging in any sort of a detox program, such as those practiced for centuries by ancient Chinese, Indian, and Native American practitioners? The answer is threefold.

First, even under ideal conditions, the body greatly benefits from periodically entering into a deeper detox mode than our everyday baseline. Think of exercise, for example. When you undertake intensive exercise, your body temporarily delays detoxification in order to fund the immense energy it needs for the exercise. Lactic acid, the by-product of intensive exercise, accumulates in the muscles until the body is once again at rest.

Similarly, eating a large meal can put detoxification on hold while the body is occupied with digesting, absorbing, and assimilating food (this is why you may feel lethargic immediately after eating a large meal!). Once exercise or digestion stops, the body is given the green light to enter a deep detox mode, by which toxins that have accumulated in the tissues can finally be released.

In our hunter-gatherer days, periods of cumulative detox happened naturally, as the unpredictable food supply meant that our ancient predecessors experienced feasts followed by famines. Without having to compete with the digestive system during these famine periods, the detox system could switch on, with plenty of time available to complete the cleanup cycles. Once we evolved into a more agrarian society and nature no longer imposed periods of fasting, healers in cultures all over the world recognized the value of coaxing our bodies into this more intensive state of detoxification through programs of fasting, diet modification, and contemplative retreats in order to reap the health benefits of the detoxification process.

Second, with the stresses and excesses of modern life, we have suppressed our bodies' detox signals to such an extent that unless we make a concerted effort, we may be overriding our natural cleanup systems to our detriment. In modern life, we rarely give our bodies enough rest for deeper detox to take place. Our cells only get the signal to release accumulated toxins when our energy reserves aren't spent on other taxing activities, but the physical, mental, and emotional demands of life in most industrialized nations are unrelenting.

Furthermore, we rarely give our digestive systems a break, as typical Western diets involve constant snacking and late-night eating. Eight hours after our last meal, our bodies are triggered to do a deep clean, which takes approximately four hours to complete. Yet few of us today allow for a full twelve-hour fast between dinner and breakfast, short-circuiting the kind of detox that's so essential to health. As a result, we may be subjecting our bodies to an excessive accumulation of toxins.

Third, not only do our bodies have to expunge their own endotoxins, but they also have to eliminate the multitude of absorbed exotoxins, the toxins introduced into our air, water, food supply, and homes since the middle of the twentieth century. Everywhere we turn, we're confronted by synthetic chemicals. Conventional factory farming relies on hormones, antibiotics, and chemical pesticides, which we, in turn, ingest in our daily meals.

As a result of global manufacturing processes, heavy metals such as mercury and arsenic have found their way into our oceans, leaving much of our seafood supply saturated with toxic levels of heavy metals. Industrially refined food additives such as high fructose corn syrup can also be contaminated with heavy metals. Automobiles and factories spew hundreds of thousands of tons of pollutants into our air every day. At home, household cleaners and cosmetics are filled with chemicals we can't even pronounce.

We've compromised our natural detox systems with our modern lifestyles of nonstop stress, constant snacking on chemical-laden convenience foods, and insufficient sleep and exercise. Add up the greater toxic load and compromised detox system, and it's clear that we're accumulating more toxins than we're expelling, putting our health in jeopardy.

Many health experts are convinced that it's no accident that so-called "diseases of civilization" have reached epidemic proportions at the same time toxins have increased and detoxification has been undermined. When our bodies do not expel as many toxins as they produce and take in, toxins remain in the tissues, where they can impede cell functioning. Over time, this can cause irritation and inflammation. This state of chronic inflammation is thought to underlie many modern diseases, including cancer, cardiovascular disease, diabetes, and auto-immune disorders.

At first, the body may show milder signs of toxicity, such as head-aches, bowel irregularities, allergies, and depression. Unfortunately, instead of treating the underlying cause of these early symptoms, many Western practitioners suppress the symptoms with drugs like antidepressants and corticosteroids, not only leaving the toxic problem unsolved, but also contributing to the body's toxic load. Over time, these minor symptoms can lead to chronic diseases that are difficult to reverse.

What is a detox program? It is any program designed to assist our bodies in drawing out, neutralizing, and eliminating toxins that have been stored in the body. It typically involves dietary and lifestyle changes aimed at reducing toxin intake, minimizing the workload of the digestive tract, and improving elimination. This may include avoiding chemicals from food and other sources, as well as avoiding refined foods, sugar, caffeine, alcohol, tobacco, and prescription drugs (whenever possible). In Ayurvedic, Chinese, and other traditional medicine programs, detoxifying herbs also play a crucial role.

There are many detox programs available to choose from today, varying from mild to extreme. Be careful: detox programs that help the body release toxins, yet do not provide enough support for neutralizing and eliminating them, can be dangerous. Some popular programs that are less intense but provide more nutritional balance include juice fasting; the water, lemon, cayenne, and maple syrup cleanse; raw food diets; and nutritional cleanses (which incorporate solid, cooked meals and soups).

The benefits of detoxification are numerous and can be difficult to quantify. In the short term, people often report improved energy, weight loss, clearer skin, more regular bowel movements, improved digestion, and increased concentration and clarity after making detox efforts. In the long term, allowing our bodies periodically to enter their natural deep cleanse mode may offer several benefits: improved immune function, reduction of chronic inflammation, and elimination of free radicals. This leaves us less vulnerable to the onset of chronic diseases.

Although I don't recommend any specific detox program as being superior to any other, I encourage you to check out two of my other books, *The Joy Factor* and *Detox & Rejuvenate*. Both offer the ultimate detox program for treating the body inside and out. They are the perfect companions to *Walking on Air*. Together they will supply you with information about healing the body, mind, and spirit to kick-start any detox program or effort you choose to undertake.

Cultivate a healthy, cleansed, and detoxified body.

∽

The sovereign invigorator of the body is exercise, and of all the exercise walking is the best.

—THOMAS JEFFERSON

Healing is a matter of time, but it is also a matter of opportunity.

—HIPPOCRATES

Today's Affirmation & Action Step

Today I fast from all negative thoughts, feelings, and emotions. I imagine my physical body filled with the restoring, loving light of Spirit. Every cell of my being is alive and revitalized with the energy of love. I feel stronger and more alive, renewed, and energized. I am healed and whole in body, mind, and spirit.

Drinking ample water supports the detoxification process. Choose to drink at least eight glasses of purified water today. Also, eat a few servings of fresh fruits and veggies because they are high in water content and provide fiber to help foster detoxification. Think of cleansing body and mind today.

Day 4

Celebrate Change and Patience

Love is an attempt to change a piece of the dream-world into reality.

—THEODOR REIK

Some men see things as they are and say "Why?" I dream of things that never were and say, "Why not?"

—GEORGE BERNARD SHAW

We live in a changing world. Nature changes constantly. Your body is different from one day to the next. Friends come and go. Feelings ebb and flow. The tide comes in and goes out. The only constant in our world is the divine. As I often say in my seminars and workshops worldwide, when the winds of change blow, go deeper—deeper within your heart.

Sometimes changes come to us as gentle breezes; other times they come as tornadoes. When changes occur, we can choose how we will respond. We can try to control and manipulate the situation. We can become upset and depressed. We can allow ourselves to be tossed around in the waves of change. Or, we can choose to dive below the surface where our strength and understanding lie.

We can remain peaceful in a changing world by aligning ourselves with our inner constancy while adapting to the passing world. Welcome change. It promotes growth and restores equilibrium by moving us in the direction of a better life awaiting us—our goals manifested. Know that when you are in harmony with your higher self, and you realize the light within you is not unlike the light in God, then in the face of all change, anything is possible.

The key here is how you respond to change. My mom helped me to look at change in my life with the proper perspective. Whenever I experienced a challenge, she would say to me, "This, too, shall pass."

Are you rigid or flexible? Being flexible is essential if you want to remain peaceful. We all have likes and dislikes. You like romantic, funny movies; your spouse likes suspense-filled, action-packed movies. You like vacationing in Hawaii, Tahiti, or France; he would prefer to tour England, Ireland, or Italy. You like fruit and a muffin for breakfast; he wants a seven-course feast. Can you feel okay that you have different tastes? Or do you get upset when you can't have your way? Be flexible! With a flexible attitude, you will float through life rather than trying to swim upstream. It's fine to have certain likes and dislikes, as long as you aren't compulsively attached to them. Be ready to change your proclivities, if necessary, as easily as you change your shoes.

It's healthy to break away from your own habits and acquiesce to another's preference. Next time your partner wants to watch a television program that doesn't interest you, view it with him and don't complain. If he wants to have Chinese food and you don't, have it anyway. Don't lose yourself in others' preferences, but be open-minded to trying out what they prefer. Train your mind to be flexible and to make the best of all situations.

Accepting change and staying open takes patience. This does not imply being unconcerned or uninterested. When we're patient, we cultivate inner peace and do not disturb the creative flow in the deep waters below. A person who is patient knows everything will unfold just as it should.

It took thousands of years for the Grand Canyon to be created. It takes a few hundred years for some redwoods to reach their full height. Relationships take time; self-improvement takes time; learning a new language takes time. Cultivate patience for all these activities and others that will reveal their eventual reward.

Let's look for a moment at your health and fitness program. Maybe at this point you are out of shape, yet you are motivated to begin exercising regularly and eating more nutritious foods. Most people don't think about all the years they've taken to get into the shape they are now. You want to see results *now*. It doesn't work that way. But with patience, determination, and perseverance, you will begin to see progress.

How do you feel around people who lack patience? The other day, I was driving with a friend to the beach. We were going to take a walk and enjoy the sunshine in Santa Monica. Our drive took us through heavy traffic. My friend got uptight, started honking the horn, and lost all his patience. I knew that wasn't exactly the best time to tell him he could choose differently, he could sit back, relax, enjoy my wonderful company (indeed!), and simply watch how all the other drivers reacted. By the time we got to the beach, his pulse was high and he couldn't relax.

Oftentimes we will be patient with others but forget to extend the same courtesy to ourselves. We make a mistake and are quick to judge and berate ourselves. When we are hurt or angry, we are seldom willing to give the situation an opportunity to reveal its lesson. We want to move through a painful situation quickly.

When we look back on our difficult or challenging situations, we find that eventually they led to greater awareness and faith. Anything worth having in life requires patience. With patience, we keep the door open to life's blessings, knowing that all is coming together for our highest good.

Celebrate change and patience today.

∼

The life given us by nature is short, but the memory of a well-spent life is eternal.

—CICERO

It is not doing the thing we like to do, but liking the thing we have to do that makes life blessed.

— JOHANN WOLFGANG VON GOETHE

Today's Affirmation & Action Step

I am patient and peaceful today, and I welcome change in my life.
Everything is working harmoniously for me, for I am a child of the Divine.
I listen patiently for the inner voice to give me guidance.

Do things differently today from your normal routine. Welcome
simple changes. For example, sleep on the opposite side of the bed, eat
a meal using a fork in your nondominant hand, take a different route
to work, or call an old friend you have not talked to for a long time
and tell that person how he or she has blessed your life. Think about
making new, positive changes today.

Day 5

Choose a Colorful, Rejuvenating Diet and Lifestyle

The supreme reality of our time is the vulnerability of our planet.

—JOHN F. KENNEDY

The wise man should consider that health is the greatest of human blessings.

—HIPPOCRATES

My reason for creating this book for you is really quite simple: I have a passion for writing—sharing my thoughts, experiences, and research on being healthy, happy, and fully alive—and a desire to help make a positive difference in people's lives. As a health researcher, writer, teacher, lecturer, counselor, and lifestyle coach for thirty-five years, I've learned that the secrets to joy and fulfillment are found in the practice of holistic health, optimal nutrition, and balanced living. My friends and clients call me "the Nature Foods Lady" and "the Nature Girl" because I always look to nature for answers.

If this is the first book of mine you have read, here's my health philosophy in a nutshell, beautifully described by Ralph Waldo Emerson: "Health is our greatest wealth." If you think about this sage advice, I'm sure you'll agree. Everything really does begin with caring about yourself. Fortunately, regardless of your current age, level of well-being, and living habits, you can choose differently at any moment. New, better choices will lead to a healthier and happier life than you ever thought possible.

If you're a baby boomer, like I am, keep in mind that changes that were once labeled milestones of growing older—such as high blood pressure, fragile bones, significant memory loss, wrinkles, reduced vision, and lack of energy and libido—are no longer considered inevitable. The diet and lifestyle choices I recommend in this book (and practice myself), and also address in my books *The Joy Factor, The Healing Power of NatureFoods, Health Bliss*, and *Recipes for Health Bliss*, will help you look and feel vibrantly alive at any age. I feel as young and exuberant as I ever did—and you can, too!

Your level of health, right this moment, is the result of the countless decisions you've made regarding your diet, exercise, thought processes, beliefs, and expectations. Undoubtedly, some of these choices may have been poor ones—but you can learn from your past mistakes. You must start, however, by making a firm commitment to your health.

True dedication begins with appreciating, respecting, and loving your magnificent body. One of the most important things you can learn in life is to appreciate yourself. As you open your heart to your own self-worth and to the divine essence of all humanity, you access the most powerful healer of all, the healing power of love. And the human body is, indeed, a miracle of Love's creation. The more I study our physical structure, the more I am amazed and in awe at how beautifully it is designed. Clearly, it's a fantastic creation that deserves reverence and respect.

Your body has a remarkable feedback system as well. If you listen, you'll discover that it actually talks to you. When you get a headache, for instance, your physical self is trying to tell you something. Make it your goal to receive its signals with health, balance, and peace. The key here is your willingness to listen and act. Start today.

Most people think that the way to handle a headache is to reach for a bottle of aspirin. While having a headache (and the countless other aches and pains that people experience) is certainly common, health is our truly normal state. Disease is an aberration, caused by harm that either you have done to yourself or others have done to you.

Collectively, Americans have made some very poor health choices. Just look at all of the commercials on television and the advertisements in magazines and newspapers. Whatever you're suffering from—headache, constipation, sleepless nights, diarrhea, indigestion, skin rashes, high blood pressure, impotency . . . fill in the blank—advertisers have a miracle pill, powder, or potion for you. We have come to believe that health and well-being can be gained from things outside us. We've become a self-medicating society because we don't really understand how beautifully robust the human body is.

I have some astonishing news for you: it's normal to be able to go to sleep at night without taking a pill; it's normal not to have headaches, sinus problems, hemorrhoids, constipation, and shaky hands. We just need to *stop doing the things that cause the problems in the first place.* When you live more from inner guidance and in a way that is closer to nature, you can enrich the quality of your life and all life on this planet. And it all begins with respecting and taking loving care of your body.

It's really not about making major lifestyle or dietary changes; rather, it's about making simple, *effective* choices that have a profound effect on your health, longevity, and quality of life. Of the many positive steps you can take, three are eminently under your control: what you eat, how much you move (physical activity), and what you think about. You have the ability to change all of these at any time. For example, you're the one who decides what you eat or drink; nobody, I hope, shoves food down your throat. If you want to be vibrantly healthy, free from disease, and filled with energy and vitality, start upgrading your choices.

Most people are digging their graves with their knives and forks. Though your diet is only one of the essential ingredients of vibrant health, it's a big one. If you're like most people, a fundamental problem is eating too many low-nutrient foods, depriving your body of the nutrients it needs. Over time, you get sick because normal functions are impaired. Even if you aren't obviously sick, you may not be healthy. Unlike a car engine, which immediately malfunctions if you put water into the gasoline tank, the human body has tremendous resilience and often camouflages the repercussions of unhealthful fuel choices. By understanding and acting on the principles of holistic nutrition described in this book, you can improve the state of your health, stave off disease, and maintain the harmonious balance that nature intended.

Walking on Air

As study after study has shown, a high-nutrient, plant-based diet is a prerequisite for optimal health. Naturally colorful foods—a rainbow of colors at each meal—are essential to help reduce your risk of heart disease, hypertension, diabetes, obesity, Alzheimer's, arthritis, common forms of cancer, premature aging, vision problems, and mental dysfunction. Foods as close to the way nature made them are the ones that are high in fiber and much-needed nutrients, and the ones that help accelerate fat loss and increase your energy level and joie de vivre.

Although eating optimal foods is important, there's more to radiant well-being than a good diet. Other essential factors must be integrated into your life if you want to maximize your health potential—and I cover these in detail in this book, *The Joy Factor*, and *Recipes for Health Bliss*.

Choose a colorful, rejuvenating diet and lifestyle today.

≈

Love yourself, heal your life.

—Louise L. Hay

Shallow men believe in luck or in circumstance. Strong men believe in cause and effect.

—Ralph Waldo Emerson

Today's Affirmation & Action Step

I am an expression of radiant health. All of life is mine to use with wisdom, joy, and delight. My health is a divine gift. I am perfect strength, and I live by nature's laws. I am in excellent health. I am whole and well. I claim my innate health and wholeness now.

Choose this day to exercise, sleep more, feel the sunshine, or spend some quality time in nature. This could be at a local park or even in your garden, especially if you have colorful flowers. Breathe deeply and think about something for which you are grateful. Think about creating your healthy lifestyle.

Day 6

Cultivate Enduring Enthusiasm and Confidence

I don't believe in failure.

—OPRAH WINFREY

Nothing great was ever achieved without enthusiasm.

—RALPH WALDO EMERSON

Many years ago, I made a decision about my work that has had great consequences. I decided that I would do only work about which I could be enthusiastic. Instead of accepting writing assignments simply because the payment was generous, I chose to write articles about which I felt great passion. It was a frightening decision for me, since at that time I lived alone and was dependent on my writing as a major source of income. But I never regretted the decision; not only did I start making more money than ever before with my chosen assignments, but I also learned a valuable lesson about enthusiasm. Enthusiasm isn't something you find out in the world; it's a God-given quality that you must choose to bring to whatever you do.

The word *enthusiasm* comes from the Greek *entheos*, meaning "to be filled with God." Isn't that fantastic? We must identify with and call forth that which is already with us. Charles Fillmore, cofounder of Unity, was in his nineties when he declared, "I fairly sizzle with zeal and enthusiasm." Regardless of our age, our line of work, or our purpose in life, we can be enthusiastic.

Dale Carnegie gave this advice: "Act enthusiastic, and you'll be enthusiastic!" In his lectures across the country and in his books, he told people not to wait for circumstances to transform their indifference into enthusiasm. "Even if you feel uninspired, act as though you were overflowing with enthusiasm," he advised. He often gave examples of people who had been failures early in life, but who persevered by having an enthusiastic outlook. Albert Einstein, Charles Darwin, and Thomas Edison all did poorly in school. Yet each possessed a great deal of enthusiasm for his work and, eventually, each one's genius became known. *When you take on an attitude—when you become it—it then becomes you.* The action itself is a kind of affirmation.

Several months of the year, I travel internationally giving workshops, seminars, and keynote addresses and doing television, radio, and newspaper interviews. One question I am asked frequently is: "How do you manage to stay so positive and enthusiastic in the face of so many local and global problems?" And I usually respond: "If I chose to be negative and unenthusiastic, that would just add to the problem. I know I can be most effective if I remain positive, optimistic, and enthusiastic."

The Bible says to be of a happy heart. I've discovered that I am the master of my life, cocreator with the Loving Presence within me. I can choose to live fully and to make a difference. Health is a choice! Happiness is a choice! Peace is a choice! And enthusiasm is the elixir that generates change, nourishes the body, and feeds the soul. As you age, your skin may become wrinkled, but without enthusiasm, your soul will wrinkle up.

A few years ago, I presented the workshop "Wellness Lifestyling" at a hospital on Oregon's southern coast. Afterward, I gave the Sunday service at a local church. While there, I met a lovely gentleman named Benny who owned and ran a bed-and-breakfast. At eighty-three years young, Benny greeted each day with enthusiasm and lots of energy. After making mouthwatering, healthy breakfasts for his clientele, he would take guests hiking, jogging, or tide-pool adventuring for a good part of the morning. After that, he would spend most of his day working on remodeling another home to which he had added a magnificent second story. When I asked him his secret for staying so enthusiastic, he responded, "Never think of your age, always look at the bright side of everything, and if something bothers you, talk it out. Don't ever hold in small grievances with a friend or spouse because they just fester and grow and create much bigger problems." I loved being around Benny because he brought out my enthusiasm and zest for life.

Enthusiasm resides in your heart—bring your heart to everything you do. Let your heart-light shine with the rays of enthusiasm permeating everything you think, feel, say, and do.

Enthusiasm and confidence are intimately connected. When you trust in something greater than yourself, enthusiasm and confidence become your natural expression. I have always admired Oprah Winfrey. No matter what, she exudes enthusiasm and confidence. She brings her heart to everything she does. And, as a result, she is successful, loved, and supported by millions of people around the world.

My favorite movie of all time is *The Sound of Music*. I've seen it more than twenty times. The governess Maria, played by Julie Andrews, personifies enthusiasm. Filled with God's presence, she radiates enthusiasm in everything she does—climbing mountains, playing with the children, singing in the abbey, or talking to God. That enthusiasm strengthens her confidence. Do you remember the song she sings called "I Have Confidence"? Its lyrics include: "I have confidence in sunshine. I have confidence in rain. I have confidence that spring will come again; besides which, you see, I have confidence in me."

With the right attitude, enthusiasm and confidence are always available. Look at everything you do as service to your Creator, as a way to do Love's work and to establish a closer relationship with your Higher Power. When your life has that purpose, you become filled with enthusiasm and confidence. The smallest tasks take on new meaning. Acknowledging and living in the presence of your inner heart-light brings peace and a whole new dimension to life.

Today, cultivate enduring enthusiasm and confidence.

~

It is better to light one small candle than to curse the darkness.

—CONFUCIUS

Enthusiasm is the mother of effort, and without it nothing great was ever accomplished. The successful person has enthusiasm.

—RALPH WALDO EMERSON

Today's Affirmation & Action Step

I greet this day with enthusiasm and confidence. It feels like I'm walking on air. With enthusiasm, I can be happy and successful at whatever I choose to do.

Today, take a normal, mundane activity and infuse it with loads of enthusiasm. If you're driving to work in bumper-to-bumper traffic, sing aloud songs that resonate in your heart. If you're doing the dishes or changing the baby's diapers, make a conscious choice to bring your enthusiastic heart into each moment of that activity. Think and act enthusiastically today no matter what you do.

Day 7

Celebrate Your Home Sanctuary

There is nothing like staying at home for real comfort.

—Jane Austen

He is the happiest, be he king or peasant, who finds peace in his home.

— Johann Wolfgang von Goethe

We all need a sanctuary in life, a place of refuge and protection, a place filled with love and peace where we can recharge our batteries and replenish our souls. For most people, this place is their home.

Do all you can to make your home a comforting place to be. As I am writing this book, I have been spending most of my time at home and have been more sensitive to my sanctuary. I notice I'm becoming less tolerant of clutter; every day I find things to give away or throw out. I feel better when my home is clean and organized.

I am also aware of how different colors influence my mood. One of my rooms is painted yellow; when I'm in that room, I feel more energetic and creative. Another one of my rooms is painted lavender; I feel more relaxed and peaceful in that room. Walk around your house and see if any of your rooms could use a face-lift. Something as simple as painting a room can make a noticeable difference.

If you have space, create a garden. It doesn't have to be elaborate. If you live in an apartment, you can have potted plants. One of the best ways to stay connected to Mother Earth is to touch her soil and nurture her plants. I rarely feel more peaceful than when I'm gardening. I love the smell of rich soil, and sitting on the ground to plant and prune. When I observe nature's beauty and order, I can't help but feel moved and inspired.

All homes are enriched by bringing nature indoors, too. Fill your home with sunlight, fresh air, and plants. Did you know that house-plants also contribute to your well-being? That's right. They provide your home with oxygen and can also clear the air of toxic chemicals. When NASA scientists placed fourteen different types of houseplants (one at a time) in a sealed Plexiglas chamber with the air pollutant benzene, they found that certain plants absorbed large amounts of this cancer-causing chemical. English ivy destroyed 90 percent of the room's benzene, while *Dracaena marginata, Dracaena* Janet Craig, peace lily, and golden pothos each had a 75 percent removal rate. Chinese ever-green absorbed half of the airborne poison. This is particularly note-worthy in light of the recent Environmental Protection Agency study showing that most of our exposure to benzene comes from indoor sources, such as cigarette smoke, latex paints, and household solvents. It won't take a jungle to clean the air you breathe indoors: NASA sci-entists estimate that one four- to twelve-inch plant per hundred square feet of floor space can dramatically reduce benzene levels.

Music is another way to bring more peace to your sanctuary. Do you ever notice how some music calms you while other music agitates you? Our bodies respond with physiological changes to different types of music. In my book *The Joy Factor,* I detail the effects of music and sound on the body, mind, and spirit and how to develop a diet of sound to achieve a calmer, more energetic, healthier self.

I'm very moved by some types of music. For example, when I listen to the old standards sung by Steve Tyrell, I always feel immediately calmer and happier. These were the songs that my mom and I always loved to listen to together. I also feel this way when I listen to Josh Groban sing-ing. The duet music of Chris Botti, composer and trumpeter, moves me in the same way, too, and makes me feel relaxed and happy. So does most music by Steven Halpern and producer David Foster. When I listen to *The Sound of Music* soundtrack, I feel uplifted and more joyful. Mozart and Bach give me energy. Heavy metal music makes me feel agitated, tense, and off-center. Next time you play music, pay close attention to how it makes you feel. I often play music featuring ocean waves, waterfalls, gentle rain, or a babbling brook. Nature's sounds create the best music for me.

A special meditation sanctuary in your home can be an extremely important place. Pick a room or a corner of a room where you'll always go when you meditate. Keep it clean, simple, and inviting. When you come to sit and commune with God, leave all else behind. I keep a special corner of my bedroom as my sanctuary, using it only for meditation. I have an altar (actually a rattan trunk) on which I placed a cover and a couple of meaningful photos, a candle, and the Bible. On the floor in front of the altar, I have a wool rug where I sit to meditate. You may prefer to sit in a chair. Because I have meditated in this corner for so many years, it contains vibrations of love and peace. When I sit to meditate, I immediately feel its calming effects.

We also need sanctuaries outside our homes, places in nature where we can go to feel safe, uplifted, empowered, and relaxed. One of my favorite places is the Self-Realization Fellowship Lake Shrine Temple in Pacific Palisades, near my home. Paramahansa Yogananda dedicated this unique sanctuary in 1950, and millions of visitors from all over the world have found inspiration in the peace and serenity that pervades these beautiful grounds. Lake Shrine is home to the Gandhi World Peace Memorial, the first monument in the world to be erected in honor of Mahatma Gandhi. Some of Gandhi's ashes are enshrined there in a thousand-year-old stone sarcophagus from China. Every time I visit Lake Shrine, I feel God's presence and leave feeling peaceful, joyful, and inspired.

I also go to a special bench on a cliff overlooking Santa Monica Bay. When I'm in town, I visit often to watch the sunset or just to think and relax. This is a special sanctuary where I can turn within to feel my connection with life and God. I feel the same way when I visit some museums, especially the Getty Museum. Place me in front of a glorious painting by a master, and I am a happy, peaceful person.

You make a place a sanctuary by bringing your intention and heart to it. Maybe there's a park, a flower garden, or a fountain down the block where you can go and sit. Perhaps you can drive to the beach, the mountains, or the desert. Find or create a special place you can visit to fill your spirit with the beauty, tranquility, and peace of nature.

Celebrate finding sanctuary today.

∼

Nothing is impossible to a willing heart.

—John Heywood

To be alive, to be able to see, to walk, to have houses, music, paintings—it's all a miracle.

—Arthur Rubinstein

Today's Affirmation & Action Step

My home is my sanctuary and is filled with the vibrations of peace and love. Everyone who visits my home feels the presence of God. I feel safe, protected, and one with the spirit of life there.

Get a new plant today that speaks to you, one that says, "I want you to take care of me, please." Maybe it will be a fragrant, colorful flower. Give it a place of honor in your home and heart. Cherish this plant and treat it with the respect it deserves. Think about beautifying your home today.

Day 8

Choose to Be CEO of Your Body and Life

I make the most of all that comes and the least of all that goes.
—SARA TEASDALE

If I've learned one thing in life, it's "Stand for something or you'll fall for anything."

—BONNIE HUNT

You are the president and CEO of your miraculous body and your life. Step up to the plate and take responsibility for this important position you have been given. High-level wellness is within your reach. Being radiantly healthy involves recognizing that all aspects of life must be integrated if you are to realize your full potential. As we learned in the last chapter, your home must be your sanctuary. So, too, your body must comfortably house your mind and your spirit. The body reflects the mind and the emotions, and the mind and the emotions reflect the spirit. For example, when your body is in good shape—fit, toned, and strong—the mind is affected positively, resulting in high self-esteem and self-confidence. The opposite is also true. The out-of-shape, sluggish, and weak body has a negative effect on the mind, which contributes to lowered self-esteem and a negative outlook on life.

The importance of health to satisfaction has always been known. As early as 300 BC, Herophilus wrote, "When health is absent, wisdom cannot reveal itself, art cannot become manifest, strength cannot be exerted, wealth is useless, and reason is powerless." In a recent Gallup survey, 75 percent of respondents rated an optimistic attitude, clean environment, stress control, good relationships, and satisfying work as very important to health. People who enjoy what they do and who feel a sense of control over their lives tend to be healthier.

Do you ever get the feeling that your life is running you, rather than you running your life? Taking charge—stepping up to your position as CEO of your body and life—means being proactive. Start with eating right and exercising regularly. These two elements can do more than add a year or two to your life span; they can improve your quality of life, especially in later years. At the end of this decade, the average life expectancy in the United States is projected to be eighty-six in some areas of the country.

Begin with your diet and exercise programs. Eat a rainbow of colorful, plant-based foods and stay active. Extensive research in the field of wellness over the past thirty-five years indicates that there are at least twenty paramount factors that must be balanced in our lives if radiant health is what we want. These include fresh air, plenty of rest and sleep, avoidance of addiction, inclusion of exercise, wholesome nutrition, sunshine, detoxification, deep breathing, a clean body, a balanced life, systematic under eating, a deep respect for life, high self-esteem, daily respites of solitude and silence, a positive attitude, a sense of belonging, and an awareness and trust in God or something bigger than your life. In this chapter, I cover a few of these briefly; the remaining are addressed in the other chapters and in my book *The Joy Factor* and my special package *Renew Your Life* available on my website. You might also enjoy the book *The Secrets of People Who Never Get Sick,* by Gene Stone. It's a marvelous and motivating book that includes practical information from a variety of people, including yours truly, about how to keep your body vibrantly healthy.

In this country, more people die of heart disease than anything else. One of the most important nutritional steps you can take to foster heart health is to manage the amount of fat in your diet. A high-fat diet is linked to heart disease and some cancers, especially of the breast, colon, and prostate. High blood pressure and stress are also linked to heart disease. Dean Ornish, MD, of the Preventative Medicine Research Institute in Sausalito, California, supervised a program for people suffering from atherosclerosis (artery blocking) and found that this condition could often be stopped and even reversed. His program (described in his book *Dr. Dean Ornish's Program for Reversing Heart Disease*) includes a low-fat vegetarian diet, yoga, breathing exercises, visualization, meditation, stress management routines, the elimination of harmful behaviors, the cultivation of a loving attitude, and moderate exercise.

For almost forty years, I have been a devotee of natural living—a wholesome diet, organic foods, fresh air and sunshine, exercise, simplicity, regular detoxification, peace of mind—which all help to keep the body healthy and clean. When you eat a healthy, colorful, nutrient-rich, high-fiber diet, this has spiritual benefits as well. Clearly, it pays to take loving care of your body, and this also includes consuming more raw foods.

Systematic under eating is essential to health and longevity. Overeating, even of healthy foods, is one of the main causes of disease and premature aging. Jesus, in the *Essene Gospel of Peace*, said, "And when you eat, never eat unto fullness." In *Spiritual Nutrition and the Rainbow Diet*, author Gabriel Cousens, MD, recommends under eating, not only for health reasons, but also for spiritual benefits. He explains that energy used for digestion is unavailable for meditation. He writes, "This is especially true if we want to get up early in the morning to meditate and we have eaten too much the night before." Scientific evidence in his book supports the efficacy of emphasizing whole, raw foods and systematically under eating for physical and spiritual rejuvenation.

Research reveals that raw foods provide the highest nutritional value and promote a natural cleansing and detoxification of the body. The energy from live foods allows your body to burn excess fat. I know this may seem hard to believe, but you can eat as much as you want and not gain weight if you eat food unaltered by processing—foods not refined, frozen, irradiated, canned, or filled with chemical preservatives. I eat lots of raw foods, and they always give me energy, make my skin glow, and build my self-esteem by giving me a feeling of well-being and being cared for. My book *The Joy Factor* has more detailed information on the benefits of raw foods and how to incorporate them into your diet.

Just as your life energy is made up of vibrations unique to you, live foods also have their own natural energy patterns. When you eat food in its original state, its life energy and yours are more easily in sync. When you eat raw nuts, your body can use their calcium and other nutrients. When you eat fresh salad greens and sprouts, your body can easily absorb their vitamins and minerals. When you eat fresh fruits, their abundant life energy imparts like energy to you.

Ancient cultures throughout the world, including the Greeks and Romans, appreciated the superior value of fruits. It has been said that the ancient Gymnosophists of India lived exclusively on fruits and vegetables. The Bible is full of references to fruits, orchards, and vineyards. One day each week for the past decade, I have eaten only fresh, raw fruit in season as a way to cleanse, rejuvenate, energize, and spiritualize my body.

Changing your eating habits can seem nearly impossible simply because likes and dislikes about food can be so rigid. Don't give food power over you. Become a master. Be the CEO of your body. From time to time, I like to let my body know who's boss by looking for opportunities to eat some special, rich, delicious food that's unhealthy and that I really want, but instead choosing something nourishing that I may not desire. When you first try this, it's hard, and your body and mind usually resist. But after a while, you feel a great sense of self-mastery, and you become free of negative impulses.

I believe that the quality of food is not the only important factor in the way we eat. The way food is prepared and served is also significant, as is the consciousness with which we eat. Food made, served, and eaten with love has a positive effect on our bodies. If we are upset, angry, agitated, or in a hurry when we eat, this affects our bodies and spirits. When we take time to appreciate our food, we support efficient assimilation of nutrients and gain a sense of satisfaction. I always meditate and say grace before a meal, even if it's only a piece of fruit. This includes thanking the Presence within and Mother Earth for these blessings of food.

We all need safe amounts of healthy sunshine, fresh air, and pure water. Air and water are sources of nutrition that the body uses to heal and renew all its cells and tissues. (Refer to my website *www.SusanSmithJones.com* and click on Favorite Products to learn more about my favorite water and purification system.) I recommend taking an air bath daily—exposing your body to fresh air and practicing deep breathing. This is especially important for those who live and work in environments that seal out fresh air. Every morning, immediately after I get up, I go out into my yard or simply open a window wide. Then I let fresh air caress by body while I participate in a variety of deep-breathing exercises. I usually do this in the evening as well. Keeping a window open while you sleep, even if it's only an inch or so in the winter, is also important. You need to breathe fresh air as much as possible. I can't emphasize enough the importance of the daily practice of deep breathing, which cleanses, detoxifies, energizes, and spiritually uplifts the body.

Rest is another important rejuvenator and healer. No magic number of hours per night works for everyone. The amount of sleep needed varies from person to person. But most of us need at least seven solid hours of good sleep nightly. Do you force yourself to stay awake to finish that one last report, clean out that one final drawer, or finish that one last chapter? If this is your regular style, watch out. A physical collapse is in the making. If you are not in good health, if you feel tired all the time and come down with frequent illnesses, if you feel too exhausted to exercise, then more extreme recuperative measures may be necessary. You may need a period of physical rest much longer than a good night's sleep. Two or three days in bed may be called for.

Exercise stimulates all the internal organs and muscle systems, tones the digestive system, rejuvenates the nerves, improves circulation, and stimulates the body and skin to release toxins. No health or rejuvenation program is complete without exercise. For those of you interested in weight loss, exercise is imperative. Your metabolic rate, which determines how many calories your body burns in its daily activities, is directly related to the amount of lean muscle mass on your body. A body with lots of metabolically active muscle burns more calories than a body that carries more fat. Exercise increases lean muscle tissue. Weight training (also called strength training), more than any other exercise, is the best way to develop lean muscle tissue. Aerobics is good for your heart and burns fat, but weight lifters use more calories all day long, even in their sleep.

When you change your lifestyle to one of wellness and rejuvenation, don't be surprised if you feel a tad worse before you begin to feel better. An initial change for the worse is often a sign that your body is doing a form of housecleaning. Your body can heal itself; you just have to supply what it needs and avoid giving it what is harmful. Balancing and supporting body, mind, and spiritual health is what will give you the feeling of walking on air. You are in charge of your body. Choose to be in alignment with nature's laws of health and healing. Persistence and commitment are the keys. Nourishing your body with fresh foods, pure water, clean air, sunshine, rest, and exercise will lead you to a level of radiance you've always dreamed of having. It's the greatest adventure imaginable.

Choose to be CEO of your body and life.

∼

To love what you do and feel that it matters—how could anything be more fun?

—KATHARINE GRAHAM

Don't judge each day by the harvest you reap but by the seeds you plant

—ROBERT LOUIS STEVENSON

Today's Affirmation & Action Step

My body is overflowing with vibrant health. I live close to nature and provide my body with everything it needs to be healthy and youthful. I choose to eat healthy, colorful foods, exercise regularly, and keep my stress levels down. All of my cells are vibrating with vitality. Each and every day, I am becoming healthier, happier, and more rejuvenated.

Take several opportunities today, perhaps at the top of the hour, for a two-to-three-minute respite of deep breathing. As you inhale and exhale slowly and deeply, focus on your miraculous body and all the ways you can give it more tender, loving care. Think healthy thoughts today.

Day 9

Cultivate the Art of Perseverance and Determination

*When faced with a mountain, I will not quit! I will keep
on striving until I climb over, find a pass through, tunnel
underneath—or simply stay and turn the mountain into a gold
mine, with God's help!*

—Robert H. Schuller

*The reason a lot of people do not recognize opportunity is
because it usually goes around wearing overalls looking like
hard work.*

—Thomas Edison

Sometimes the answer to a challenge or the guidance that we seek
seems just beyond our reach. This is the time to keep on keeping
on. You can win the race no matter how far behind you are when you
start. Keep your goal clearly in sight, and don't get sidetracked.

Life can be complicated. It's easy to lose sight of our purpose in the
midst of our daily lives. We often become wrapped up in the demands
of our schedules, paying the bills, rearing children, or getting ahead
at work. We live our lives from a rabbit's-eye view—our noses pressed
up against the blade of grass right in front of us. Just as grasping the
beauty of an entire tapestry is difficult if we view it too closely, we can,
similarly, lose clarity. We must learn to take an eagle's-eye view. Soaring

far above the ground, the eagle can see farther and with greater clarity than the earthbound rabbit. And as the eagle uses the wind to keep it aloft, you can choose to use determination and perseverance to keep yourself on course.

Recently, I read *The Big Book of Women Saints,* by Sarah Gallick, and was fascinated by Saint Teresa of Avila, also known as Saint Teresa of Jesus. She grew up in the sixteenth-century Spanish town of Avila and was intelligent, beautiful, sagacious, and charming. While she was still a teen, she began to realize that the things of the world did not have nearly so much appeal for her as the things of the spirit. She prayed for greater awareness, clarity, and strength to follow her heart. What was it that made her listen to her heart and follow that guidance? Determination. It's one of the qualities she emphasized. "Those who have this determination," she revealed, "have nothing to fear."

How determined are you to live joyfully, healthfully, and peacefully? How determined are you to keep on going when the going gets tough? When I began writing, approximately thirty years ago, I received more than a hundred rejection letters from magazines. There were times I felt like giving up. Even my close friends and some family members encouraged me to seek another profession. "You can't pay your bills on dreams," they would tell me. "Look for a job that offers security, a regular monthly paycheck, and normal hours," was something I heard regularly. Well, I'm glad to say I didn't listen to them. I was determined to be true to my vision and dreams. Now many years later, I've written more than twenty-seven books and over 1,500 magazine articles. Editors now approach me to write articles for their magazines. Determination and perseverance always pay off.

I love the following words that appear in Richard Bach's insightful book, *Illusions:* "You are never given a wish without also being given the power to make it true. You may have to work for it, however."

I have great respect for world-class athletes who, against all odds, become winners. And I'll never forget the story about the cyclist Greg LeMond. In 1985, he finished second in the arduous Tour de France, a twenty-three-day 2,025-mile cycling race through France. Then in 1986, at the age of twenty-five, LeMond became the first non-European ever to win the race. With his prime competitive years still ahead of him, Greg LeMond was on top of the world.

Within a few months, however, his life turned upside down. In April 1987, LeMond was with his uncle and his brother-in-law on a hunting trip when he was hit by a shotgun blast. His brother-in-law had accidentally shot him. LeMond took approximately sixty No. 2 pellets in his back and side. He could barely breathe; his right lung had collapsed. His liver and kidney were hit. So were his diaphragm and intestines. And two pellets were lodged in the lining of his heart. LeMond thought he was going to die as he lay in the field waiting for the helicopter that would take him to the hospital. His main concern was whether he would ever see his wife and kids again.

While in the hospital, LeMond learned about real pain. A tube to draw blood out of his collapsed lung had to be inserted into his chest without anesthesia, and it remained there for a week. He had thought he was accustomed to pain because he had pushed himself so hard in competition. But the pain he felt while racing his bike was nothing compared with the pain he felt as he fought for his life.

Doctors left thirty shotgun pellets in LeMond, including the two in the lining of his heart. They doubted that LeMond would ever race again. Eight weeks later, however, with sheer determination and perseverance, he started the long road back. Before the accident, LeMond weighed 151 pounds, with a total body fat content of 4 percent. When he was able to start training again, he weighted 137 pounds, with 17 percent body fat. In an effort to survive, his body had consumed vast amounts of its own muscle.

He had a rough two years coming back. Months after the accident, just when he was beginning to show signs of real progress, he had an emergency appendectomy. The following year, he had to have surgery to repair an infected tendon in his right shin, forcing him to miss the Tour de France for a second straight year. PDM, the Dutch team with which LeMond had signed a two-year deal in 1987, wanted to cut his 1989 salary by $200,000. The team had lost all confidence in him. But he had not lost confidence in himself. LeMond entered the 1989 Tour de France, along with 155 other riders, and came out the winner. Determination makes all things possible.

Are you willing to do what it takes to become master of your life? Do you have the sheer will to give it your all, and then some, even when the odds of attaining your goal appear to be insurmountable? As a cocreator with God, you have the power and ability to achieve your heart's desire. Let your perseverance and determination fuel your mind and body into action. Know that the Loving Presence within you is your strength and power. When you feel that connection, peace will be your constant companion, and success will be yours.

Cultivate the art of perseverance and determination today.

~

People seldom see the halting and painful steps by which the most insignificant success is achieved.

—ANNIE SULLIVAN

Perseverance is more prevailing than violence, and many things that cannot be overcome when they are together, yield themselves up when taken little by little.

—PLUTARCH

Today's Affirmation & Action Step

I keep my sights focused on my goal and refuse to be discouraged. Divine love, flowing through me, gives me the strength and determination to follow my heart and achieve my heart's desires. I will persevere, for I know my success is assured. Anything is possible if I trust and believe.

During your exercise session today, just when you think you can't push any harder, push forward for another ninety seconds to two minutes. Or if you have no plans to exercise, do it. Even if you're in your office, you can step in place for ten minutes. Running errands? Park at the far corner of the parking lot. Take the stairs instead of the elevator or the escalator and climb—don't stand still on the moving ramp. Think about taking action and doing your best today.

Day 10

Celebrate Nature's Wonderland
of Healing Herbs and Spices

*The doctor of the future will no longer treat the human frame
with drugs, but rather will cure and prevent disease with
nutrition.*

—THOMAS EDISON

*Is not birth, beauty, good shape, discourse, manhood, learning,
gentleness, virtue, youth, liberality, and such like the spice and
salt that season a man?*

—WILLIAM SHAKESPEARE

It could be said that the history of the modern world was created in pursuit of spices. The desire of Europeans and Arabs for exotic flavorings, nearly all of which originated in Asia, sowed the seeds of modern globalization.

The Egyptians were the first to initiate the spice trade, importing cassia and cinnamon from China and Southeast Asia as far back as 1550 BC. For hundreds of years, Arab merchants sustained a monopoly over the delivery of spices as valuable as gold from the Orient to Europe. When the fall of the Roman Empire in 641 AD severed spice trade routes along the Silk Road between India and the Mediterranean, powerful Western European nations scrambled to find a maritime shortcut. This lust for spices motivated Columbus to set sail for India in the fifteenth century, when he found the New World, and led the British, Dutch, Spanish, and Portuguese to compete heatedly for control of newly discovered spice lands in the Americas.

You may be wondering, what was all the fuss about? With a cornucopia of spices readily available at our local grocery stores, it's hard to imagine a time when spices were a scarce luxury only the very wealthy could afford. Throughout the history of the spice trade, spices were prized for the unparalleled depth of flavoring they lent to food. They were also imbued with metaphysical value. Egyptians used aromatic spices in the embalming process to ward off evil, while European Christians thought exotic plants such as cinnamon were the scents of paradise.

But perhaps most important, the curative potential of spices was recognized from the earliest of times. Ancient Egyptian physicians used spices for medicinal purposes. In ancient Greece, Hippocrates, the father of modern medicine, wrote treatises on the healing properties of spices such as saffron, cinnamon, thyme, mint, and marjoram.

Today, science is affirming that spices have antioxidant, antimicrobial, and anti-inflammatory properties. Furthermore, spices may aid in the prevention and treatment of a host of diseases both minor and serious, ranging from the discomfort of colds and flu to arthritis and heart disease. In reaching for remedies from the spice rack rather than the medicine cabinet, we not only avoid many of the unfavorable side effects of pharmaceuticals, we can also reconnect with the traditions of our ancestors.

As mentioned in the introduction, my own grandmother Fritzie taught me how to take care of my body inside and out using only natural remedies. My entire pantry is filled with natural remedies that I use personally and in my private practice.

So, what exactly is a spice? Spices are often linked with their close companions, herbs, but there are important distinctions between the two. While herbs are typically the leaves of plants, spices originate from a plant's aromatic parts, including the root (e.g., ginger), the bark (e.g., cinnamon), the flower (e.g., saffron), the berries (e.g., peppercorn), and the seed (e.g., cumin). Herbs are at their most potent and flavorful when fresh, but most spices gain their flavor and healing properties in the drying process, when naturally occurring enzymes are activated. Fortunately, that means you can keep a selection of spices at your fingertips year-round.

Following is a list of some spices you have probably used in your cooking but may not know can also be used as medicine.

Black Pepper—This everyday spice appears to produce changes that can reduce the severity of seizures in the brains of mice. Have a minor cut? Sprinkle some freshly ground black pepper on it. I mix it into a paste with aloe vera gel and put it directly on the cut. It helps stop the bleeding quickly. You'll be surprised by how well this works. It doesn't sting or burn, and it actually reduces the pain and even has antibacterial and antiseptic properties. Extra bonus: it helps prevent scarring.

Cinnamon—This spice is a valuable commodity. In fact, in some ancient cultures, it was once considered more valuable than gold! Today, it is still valued as a tasty spice, but it is also now appreciated for the natural compounds it contains.

Cinnamon improves your body's ability to manage insulin production, thereby effectively breaking down and absorbing glucose (blood sugar). It also cuts heart-threatening triglycerides and bad low-density lipoprotein (LDL) cholesterol. Cinnamon helps mollify inflammation and is a time-honored digestive aid. If one of my clients calls me with an upset stomach or wants advice on how to relieve gas and bloating, I often suggest cinnamon. I take cinnamon in capsule form daily. It's a warming, circulatory tonic that increases blood flow throughout the body.

Top tip: Sprinkle cinnamon on your morning coffee, toast, or oatmeal. You could also double the amount you use in recipes for baked foods, sprinkle it on baked sweet potatoes, add it to chili and curries for authentic flavor, or create a zero-carb, flavorful, and refreshing drink by adding a cinnamon stick to your glass or bottle of water (it should last for two days).

Cloves—A compound in cloves called eugenol is a powerful inflammation fighter and a popular numbing compound found in many products used by dentists during root canal surgery. It may even help cut the risk of digestive system cancers.

Fenugreek—These aromatic seeds, which are used in curry powder, contain compounds called saponins, which bind to cholesterol and cause it to be excreted from the body. In one study, scientists found that animals given fenugreek had drops in cholesterol of at least 18 percent.

Garlic—In ancient Greece and Rome, athletes ate garlic before competitions and soldiers consumed it before battle. Today, science has proven the many ways in which garlic reinforces our vigor and vitality. First and foremost, garlic is a triple threat (and treat!) when it comes to cardiovascular health. Numerous studies have shown that regular consumption of garlic can lower blood pressure, inhibit coronary artery calcification, and decrease platelet aggregation, thereby reducing the risk of blood clots and coronary artery disease. It can also prevent the oxidation of cholesterol in the bloodstream that leads to heart disease.

Allicin, a sulfur compound found in garlic, is a powerful antibacterial, antiviral, and antifungal capable of killing harmful microbes, making garlic a natural antidote to colds, flu, and infections. Research shows that garlic can stop the *H. pylori* bacterium (associated with stomach ulcers and cancer) from doing excessive damage. Eating as little as two servings of garlic a week reduces the risk of colon cancer significantly. For forty years, I've supplemented my diet with Kyolic Aged Garlic Extract. For a free sample of Kyolic or other Wakunaga of America products (availability varies), please call: 1-800-421-2998 or visit: *www.Kyolic.com.* (Visit Favorite Products on my website *www. SusanSmithJones.com* for more information on this stellar nutritional supplement.)

Ginger—This root is used by billions worldwide. And no wonder! This aromatic spice invigorates healthy digestion, boosts circulation, and is an effective warming digestive and circulatory tonic. It's my favorite go-to remedy for the prevention and treatment of nausea and vomiting associated with motion sickness. (When I fly, I take capsules hourly to prevent motion sickness. It's good when driving, too.) One study involving eighty naval cadets revealed that 1,000 milligrams of ginger powder capsules controlled symptoms including nausea, vomiting, vertigo, and cold sweats. Most mornings, I make a hot beverage of purified water and fresh ginger.

A compound in ginger called gingerol has a chemical structure somewhat similar to aspirin, which is a proven clot-busting drug. There's also growing evidence that ginger can help quell the inflammation associated with some forms of arthritis. The gingerol in ginger relaxes blood vessels and helps calm the body.

Red Hot Cayenne—This spice shows promise for cutting cancer risk due to the anti-inflammatory and antioxidant properties of the compound capsaicin. There's a saying "Whatever doesn't kill you, makes you stronger." These thermogenic morsels are prized for their healing power and their firepower.

Hot chilies or cayenne powder, research suggests, may also help you win the battle of the bulge. Cayenne provides a three-pronged attack against obesity. First, eating cayenne may help fight off food cravings. Some experts believe that eating sharp-tasting foods such as hot peppers can overwhelm taste buds, cutting off cravings. Second, cayenne helps you eat less. Researchers in the Netherlands gave men 0.9 grams of ground cayenne pepper, either as a pill or mixed into a tomato juice beverage. Then thirty minutes later, they turned the men loose at an all-you-can-eat buffet. Compared with men who were given a placebo, those who had consumed cayenne reduced their food intake by up to 16 percent. Third, it actually requires energy to eat hot peppers. That's right—eating hot peppers burns calories. The heat you feel when you eat them takes energy to produce. That's why I've added cayenne capsules to my daily health and nutrition program.

Rosemary—You may have heard the old saying "Rosemary is for remembrance." Rosemary is full of antioxidants that will help keep your memory sharp and is excellent for overall mental health. This pungent herb can enhance your sauces and liven up breads and muffins. A tiny bit goes a long way, so start with a minimal amount. You can always add more. When you reach for your seasonings, remember rosemary.

Saffron—Compounds from saffron were placed on human cancer cells, as well as cells that cause leukemia. Not only did the dangerous cells stop growing, but the normal, healthy cells appeared to be unaffected by the compounds.

Sage—To be sage means to possess wisdom, and you would certainly be wise to incorporate this native Mediterranean spice into your diet. Research shows that sage can enhance memory and guard against the development of Alzheimer's disease. In fact, Chinese sage contains compounds similar to those found in modern drugs used to treat Alzheimer's disease.

Like rosemary, sage is a source of rosmarinic acid, an antioxidant known to protect cells from free radical damage and to reduce inflammation, making sage beneficial for arthritis sufferers. Sage tea has traditionally been used as a digestive aid, which quickly relieves gas and soothes an upset stomach. Its naturally occurring essential oils calm and relax muscle cramps and spasms.

Sage is a smart accompaniment to turkey and stuffing, bean dishes, and baked squash. It adds warm, wonderful flavor to seafood, vegetables, and breads. You may even burn sage leaves as incense to freshen the air.

Turmeric—This spice is best known as the aromatic ingredient that gives curry its vibrant, golden color. Medicinally, it's recognized as a powerful antioxidant and shows promise in maintaining healthy cholesterol levels. It has one of the highest known sources of beta-carotene. In my private practice, I highly recommend turmeric to help reduce inflammation, support healthy joint function, and relieve aching joints. You can add this spicy powerhouse to your life either in capsules, liquid extract, or as a powdered spice.

Turmeric is also a rich source of curcumin, which has been shown to reduce the risk of colon cancer by 58 percent in animal studies. Curcumin has also been shown to protect the eyes from free radicals, which are one of the leading causes of cataracts. Other studies have found that curcumin supplement could ease the pain and inflammation of rheumatoid arthritis and other inflammatory conditions. In fact, when people with AIDS were given curcumin (inflammation generally increases in AIDS patients), the illness progressed at a slower rate.

For more information on the healing power of spices and herbs, please visit my website *www.SusanSmithJones.com*, click on Natural

Remedies, and check out the series of booklet/CD combos. For decades, I have purchased herbs, spices and seasonings, and other natural remedies through the Penn Herb Company. They have over 7,000 products to choose from at *www.PennHerb.com*. You'll also want to visit *www. SusansRemedies.com*.

Celebrate nature's wonderland of healing herbs and spices today.

~

To sit in the shade on a fine day and look upon verdure is the most perfect refreshment.

—Jane Austen

When we focus on what we love, we fashion our life around our inner knowledge. We live the life we choose, surrounding ourselves with people we love and objects that hold great meaning. Home is a good place to begin our concentration because it is our emotional center. Then we can branch out in all directions, spreading the light of our true essence and heart's desire.

—Alexandra Stoddard

Today's Affirmation & Action Step

I celebrate nature's wonderland of herbs and spices. My meals are always satisfying and filled with nutrients galore. I spice up my life every day with these gems of nature.

If you don't have any on hand, get some cinnamon sticks today and put one in your water. Transfer it from glass to glass and bottle to bottle. Cinnamon is great for anyone who wants to have more energy, desires to look younger, has a tummy ache, or wants balanced blood sugar.

Day 11

Choose to Organize and Simplify Your Surroundings

The simplification of life is one of the steps to inner peace. A persistent simplification will create an inner and outer well-being that places harmony in one's life.

—PEACE PILGRIM

Simplify! What a wonderful word and a powerful process. As part of my rejuvenation makeover program, I am simplifying my life—not just my home environment, but also every aspect of my life. It is such a freeing experience. Every day I do something to unclutter my life—clean a drawer or closet, give away some possessions, or spend time just sitting and watching the birds outside my window as a way to simplify how I'm using my time—doing one thing wholeheartedly. As you know from my previous chapters, making your home a sanctuary is essential to achieving a new level of inner peace. Make simplifying and beautifying your surroundings part of this process.

The death of a dear friend recently made me sit down and think about life and about how I could choose to live more fully. The following words by Alfred D'Souze came to mind:

> For a long time it had seemed to me that life was
> about to begin—real life. But there was always some
> obstacle in the way, something to be got through

first, some unfinished business, time still to be served,
a debt to be paid. Then life would begin. At last it
dawned on me that these obstacles were my life.

This reminded me that sometimes our lives are so cluttered, it's difficult to see clearly. We are all trying to orchestrate the complexities and responsibilities of our modern lives. As we grow in self-awareness and live more intentionally, life gets simpler. Instead of getting our cues from the outside world, we listen for cues from our hearts.

Simplifying doesn't necessarily mean we have to restrict our activities, but it does mean uncluttering our lives so that we can put all our energy into activities we really care about. Activities, material things, and relationships are all time and energy consumers. It's time to take inventory of your life and weed out the superfluous. Being clear allows us to experience the present more fully and deeply.

Plato wrote, "In order to seek one's own direction, one must simplify the mechanics of ordinary, everyday life." To begin uncluttering your life, start with your home. Weed out everything you don't need, want, and use. Spend fifteen minutes a day working on one area of your home, like a drawer or a closet. After your home is simplified, look at how you live, what you do, and how you spend your time. For example, look at all the foods you eat in one meal. It's hard to appreciate any one of them fully when there are so many at once. Similarly, you could have a fantastic collection of art objects in your home, but if there are too many, it can be difficult to appreciate each piece fully. By the same token, if you have too many obligations, details, and responsibilities, life loses its luster.

This theme of simplicity runs through many great spiritual teachings. Saint Francis of Assisi is known for embracing a life of simplicity. (A movie I enjoy, available on DVD, is *Brother Sun, Sister Moon,* about simplicity and the life of Saint Francis.) Another one of my favorites is Brother Lawrence, who discovered and wrote about the power of living a life of simplicity; he saw God in the most mundane expressions of life. In *Practicing the Presence,* he wrote, "I began to live as if there was none but He and I in the world."

Walking on Air

Peace Pilgrim was another personification of simplicity. To the world, she may have seemed poor, being penniless and wearing her only material possessions. But she was rich in blessings that no amount of money could buy—health, happiness, and inner peace. The quality of our lives isn't created outside ourselves. It comes from a healthy self-image, serenity, and our relationship with the loving light within us. Peace Pilgrim wrote:

> The simplified life is a sanctified life,
> Much more calm, much less strife.
> Oh, what wondrous truths are unveiled—
> Projects succeed which had previously failed.
> Oh, how beautiful life can be.
> Beautiful simplicity.

One of the greatest lessons Peace Pilgrim taught me was to simplify outer things so that my inner life can take the driver's seat. Living an uncluttered life gives me time for the things I really care about; I am a more clear-minded and, I believe, kinder, more sensitive person. When there is time to meditate, walk, read, reflect, think, pray, and be in the simplicity and beauty of nature, then life has a more natural flow.

There seems to be a trend toward simplicity these days. Stanford Research Institute social scientist Duane Elgin points out in *Voluntary Simplicity:*

> To live with simplicity is to unburden our lives—to
> live a more direct, unpretentious, and unencumbered
> relationship with all aspects of our lives: consuming,
> working, learning, relating, and so on. Simplicity
> of living means meeting life face to face. It means
> confronting life clearly, without unnecessary
> distractions, without trying to soften the awesomeness
> of our existence or masking the deeper manifestations
> of life with pretensions, distractions, and unnecessary
> accumulations. It means being direct and honest in
> relationships of all kinds. It means taking life as it is. . . .

That passage really rings true for me. Letting go of the clutter, living honestly, simply and freely, without pretensions, encumbrances, and superfluity is what living fully is all about. Perhaps we can head in that direction by having fewer desires and being more selfless. The venerable Lao-Tzu said:

> Manifest plainness
> Embrace simplicity
> Reduce selfishness
> Have few desires.

Having fewer desires starts with being happy with and grateful for what you have. After Gandhi met with the King of England, a reporter commented on how scantily dressed he had been in the presence of the king. Gandhi replied, "It's okay. The king has on enough for both of us."

There was a time in my life when I found great pleasure in collecting material things. I would delight in buying lots of clothes, shoes, accessories, appliances, electronics, gadgets, and cars until I got to the point where I was seeking fulfillment from what I collected rather than from within. In the pursuit of material possessions, I began to lose sight of the spiritual side of my nature, through which all fulfillment, joy, peace, and happiness come. I was looking outward, to my collection of things, for my value and worthiness as a human being rather than looking within.

Fortunately, I discovered it's not what the world holds for you that is important, but what you bring to the world. When I realized that, it became clear to me that I wanted to live more simply. Sure, I still buy clothes and other items, but more often I'm giving away things and finding ways to make my life less complicated.

When we have chaos in our lives, including in our homes, we feel chaotic in our minds. Here is a ritual I've kept for years. I invite a friend over to my house weekly for a cup of tea, a homemade treat, and a special visit; it helps motivate me to clean my home and to consistently get rid of clutter and the nonessentials.

I want to close by sharing with you a passage I read a few days ago in the book *The Simple Life*, by Joan Atwater.

Our lives are over-burdened, and living often seems to us a terribly complicated affair. The problems of the world are so incredibly complex and we see that there are no simple answers. The complexity always leaves us with a feeling of helplessness and powerlessness. And still, amazingly enough, we go on, day by day, always half subconsciously yearning for something simpler, something more meaningful.

So how we look at our lives and living becomes tremendously important. It's up to us to bring this authenticity, this simplicity, this directness, this unburdened clarity into our looking. If such a thing as living life fully interests you, then it's up to you to learn about it and live it.

Choose to organize and simplify your surroundings.

~

Simply being alive is the greatest blessing we can enjoy.
—René Dubos

Our life is frittered away by detail . . . Simplify, simplify.
—Henry David Thoreau

Today's Affirmation & Action Step

I become as a little child today with my arms outstretched to touch life's simple pleasures. Miracles abound in my life, and I lift my awareness to see and attract miracles to me. I dwell in joy, and I live simply so that I may live in harmony and alignment with the peace that underlies all life.

Take at least fifteen minutes today to search your home for items you no longer need and you can give to someone or some organization that can use them. Think about decluttering today.

Day 12

Cultivate a Tender Heart and Loving Kindness

Only a life lived for others is worth living.

—Albert Einstein

What do we live for, if not to make life easier for each other?

—George Eliot

Gentleness and kindness are usually in tandem. The word *gentle* means to be kindly, mild, amiable, and not violent or severe. It means being compassionate, considerate, tolerant, calm, mild-tempered, courteous, and peaceful. But I think that the best synonym for being gentle is tenderhearted. I love that word. And I love being around people who are tenderhearted.

To be treated with tenderheartedness, we must first offer this quality to other people. Respond to others exactly as you would want to be treated. No one likes to be rushed or belittled, ignored or unappreciated. Ephesians 4:32 advises, "Be kind to one another, tenderhearted, forgiving one another." And throughout the Gospels, Jesus teaches, "As you have believed, so let it be done unto you" (Matt. 8:13).

Reaching out with a kind act or word of praise or appreciation can be so simple. Yet sometimes we assume that others have it together, and do not need our kindness. Wouldn't it be better to move beyond our assumptions and to offer the kind of thoughtfulness we appreciate receiving—a compliment, a smile, a hug, a pat on the shoulder, a note of thanks, or just a question that shows concern? If your kind gesture goes unnoticed or is refused, it doesn't matter, because in giving to another, you give to yourself. You'll feel better. Gandhi said that the pure loving kindness of one gentle soul could nullify the hatred of millions. Now is the time for all of us to live more tenderheartedly.

Think about the power of smiling. Everyone can do it. It takes seventeen muscles to smile and forty-seven muscles to frown. It's so simple, and yet so effective. Learn to smile sincerely, from your heart. No matter the circumstance, no matter how challenging the situation, put on a happy face. Smile to family and friends, to strangers, to everyone you meet or pass during the day. Do you realize how many lives you can touch simply by smiling? Smiling transmits good feelings that the other person will catch and then use to smile at another person, and so on, until your smile has, indirectly, affected the lives of several thousand people in one day.

How about writing a note of thanks? A real note, sent in the postal mail, rather than through e-mail. It doesn't take much time. Sending notes is becoming a lost art form, and it's such a simple, considerate act of kindness. I learned about this from my dear friend Alexandra Stoddard whose wonderful, heart-stirring book *Gift of a Letter* changed my life. I love to write letters and notes and am very faithful, as most of my friends will attest. Sometimes I'll go to a card store and purchase several dozen cards to have on hand. Isn't it fun to receive a card from a friend for no reason at all?

Another act of kindness I always appreciate is a hug or simply the touch of another person. Since I was a young girl, my mom, June (who passed away last decade), was always my shining example on how to treat others with kindness. She encouraged me to be loving and kind to others, to offer a gentle yet appropriate touch to another, such as on the shoulder or arm, or even a thoughtful hug. She would always repeat her prescription to health and happiness: "to keep the doctor away, give five hugs each day." I've been known to give hugs in important business meetings, even when I've just met the person. I've had my share of awkward looks, but it's how I like to be, and unless someone specifically says to me that he doesn't like to be touched, I will continue following my heart and doing what feels right to me.

Touching does so much. Studies at the University of Colorado Medical School have shown that touching increases hemoglobin, increases immune functioning, decreases tension in the body, and accelerates healing. Yes, there is great power in our hands.

Recently, I visited a friend in the hospital. When I walked into her room, she began complaining about her male nurse acting forgetful and rude. When my friend left the room for her therapy, her nurse came in to change the sheets. I could see the pain and anguish on his face, so I offered a few kind words about how much I appreciated his hard work and dedication. That opened the way for him to reveal the incredible hardship in his life. His wife still lived in South Africa and his two children had recently died from medical complications. He was working a double shift just to make ends meet. When I heard all this, I felt a deep, loving kindness for him. Before he left the room, I gave him a big hug. He started to cry. You know how that can be sometimes? All it takes is a hug or a kind word and the emotional floodgates open.

Over the next couple weeks, whenever I visited my friend, I took the nurse some of my homemade organic granola, muffins, cupcakes, cookies, or bread, which he loved and appreciated. Both my hospitalized friend and I learned a valuable lesson during those two weeks about how important it is to reach out to others with tenderheartedness even though you have no guarantee of what you'll get in return.

Sometimes the kindest gestures can go unnoticed. I love to put coins in parking meters when I walk down the street if I find some that have expired. The drivers of the cars never know what I have done, but it makes me feel good. Sometimes I send a note anonymously with a kind word or a few dollars when I know the recipient is in need. It takes so little to contribute, and you receive so much in return.

Each of us can make a difference in the world. It is a strong person who is gentle. We always feel at peace with such a person. When we relax and are centered in the divine flow, we express this gentle kindness toward ourselves and toward others.

To be gentle and kind to others, we must first be gentle and kind with ourselves. There's no need to be hard on yourself when you make a mistake. Just as God forgives us, we must forgive ourselves. Through love and forgiveness, we can live from our hearts and live in the heart of Love. And when we live in the heart of Love, of God, we can let our tenderheartedness shine through in everything we think, feel, say, and do.

Cultivate a tender heart and loving kindness.

~

To have peace and confidence within our souls—these are the beliefs that make for happiness.

—MAURICE MAETERLINCK

Kindness is the language we all understand. Even the blind can see it and the deaf can hear it.

—MOTHER TERESA

Today's Affirmation & Action Step

Peacefully and gently, I relax and feel the love in my heart. I let go of any thoughts of unkindness or unforgiveness toward myself and others. In everything I think, feel, say, and do, I let my gentleness and my kindness shine through.

Send a note of kindness to someone today for no reason at all except to say, "I appreciate you. You bless and enrich my life." While you're at it, send a love note to yourself, too. Think only loving, kind thoughts today.

Day 13

Celebrate the Power of the Present

The ability to be in the present moment is a major component of mental wellness.

—ABRAHAM MASLOW

Every situation—no, every moment—is of infinite worth; for it is the representative of a whole eternity.

— JOHANN WOLFGANG VON GOETHE

Living *in* the moment is different from living *for* the moment. Children seem to be the masters of living in the moment, of being able to be totally engrossed in whatever they are doing. When they eat, they just eat; when they play, they just play; when they talk, they just talk. They throw themselves wholeheartedly into every activity.

I look back on my early childhood and remember not having any sense of time. My family frequently took long trips in the car. Usually within ten minutes of leaving, I would ask, "Are we there yet?" My only sense of time was now. It was sheer joy to have my family all together in the car taking trips to wonderful destinations. Seneca said, "True happiness is to . . . enjoy the present, without anxious dependence upon the future." As a child, I instinctively knew this, especially when I was with my family.

Carpe diem. That's Latin for "seize the day." Each day offers us an opportunity to look at the world anew and to celebrate being alive. You'll never have an opportunity to live this precious day again. Moment by moment, choose to be aware of everything around you. Notice the flowers, the air, your family pets, babies, the sunrise and sunset, the stars. Breathe in the radiance of these glorious miracles.

Have you ever noticed that young children are willing to try anything at a moment's notice? Even though they might have experienced the same thing before, they will express wide-eyed excitement and wonderment. Children don't use a yardstick to measure activities or compare the present with the past. They know they've played the game before, or had someone read the same story just last night, yet the game or the story is still as fresh and as wonderful as it was the first time.

Think about your attitude when doing the dishes, vacuuming, or watering the plants. You probably find these activities boring. Have you ever seen a child help with the dishes or vacuum or water the plants? A child acts as though it's just about the most exciting thing she has ever done. What a wonderful quality that is! It's only old thoughts and distorted attitudes that get in the way of celebrating each moment.

Often when I'm conducting a workshop or seminar in a beautiful, natural setting somewhere around the world, I ask the participants to go outside for ten to fifteen minutes, breathe deeply, and stroll the grounds, alone, in silence. I have them practice being totally absorbed in what they see, smell, taste, feel, and hear. To be with nature, letting its beauty into your awareness, is a wonderful experience. In taking this kind of walk, I have discovered that I feel a subtle, gentle communion with nature. The flowers, trees, birds—even the insects—seem to be in harmony with me.

Most people work so hard at living that they forget how to life fully in the moment. When you give the present moment a chance to infuse your mind and heart, the glorious and serendipitous can blossom. Give the unexpected a chance to bloom through present-moment awareness combined with deep breathing.

Do your best each day to simplify your life, and to value and experience the preciousness of nature and every moment. Rather than living with continual five- or ten-year plans, concentrate on living one day at a time, continuing to ask for guidance and direction each day. I ask my guardian angels daily to guide me and to bring more light and miracles my way. Don't look back in anger or regret, or forward in fear or worry, but look around with conscious awareness and gratitude. George Gershwin, one of my favorite American composers and pianists, wrote, "My time is today."

To be fully present each moment, free yourself from the past. Otherwise, the past will repeat itself and keep you trapped in it, as I write about in detail in my book *The Joy Factor* and cover in *Renew Your Life*, my 14-title compendium which is available on my website. When you're trapped in the past, you're not fully aware of the present, you can't see what's happening all around you.

No matter what issues you are dealing with, the road to healing begins with a gentle step inward to seek the heart-light within. We must be gentle with ourselves and, with divine help, courageous. The shadow side of our nature is what we've hidden from ourselves out of fear. It is a repository filled with long-forgotten tears, secret anguish and pain, abdicated power, and thwarted dreams. It's the locked-away part of your soul. Your shadow is not itself dark, but it is hidden in a dark place where you have feared to go. You must take that step. If you feel it's too difficult to do on your own, seek help.

One of the splendors of being human is our capacity to learn from mistakes. Don't let your fear hold you back. "I saw that all things I feared, and which feared me, had nothing good or bad in them save insofar as the mind was affected by them," wrote Spinoza. When you let go of fear, pain will unfold into joy, sadness will unfold into happiness, and hate will turn into love.

When you heal your past, your life will take on a new sense of wonder and celebration. You will become more aware of yourself and everything around you. When you live in the present, breathe deeply, and keep awareness, you can live with heart, knowing that the love you are is all that is needed. You will find yourself immersed in wisdom and peace and one with the Infinite. Isn't that what living is all about? Don't wait any longer. Now is the time. Trust more.

Choose to celebrate the present moment.

≈

Write it on your heart that every day is the best day of the year.

—RALPH WALDO EMERSON

All moments are key moments, and life itself is grace.

—FREDERICK BUECHNER

Today's Affirmation & Action Step

I choose to live each moment to the fullest, one day at a time. I let go of the past and know that my future will be bright and happy because I live from love, trust, and faith. Divine order is taking place in my life right now.

Find five to fifteen minutes today to be by yourself. Whether in your home or office, or in your car or a place in nature, choose to be still, breathe deeply, keep your focus and attention on the present moment, and feel deep gratitude for your life. Think about dwelling in the present moment today.

Day 14

Choose to Be Self-Disciplined

*To act magnanimously, to maintain high standards, to be
honorable, requires commitment to yourself. Make it.*
—ALEXANDRA STODDARD

*Character isn't inherited. One builds it daily by the way one
thinks and acts, thought by thought, action by action.*
—HELEN GAHAGAN DOUGLAS

Discipline is a choice. If we are to live our highest potential, the
way we were all created to be, we must practice self-discipline in
every aspect of our lives. It's the only way to live on higher ground. The
mountain of soul-achievement and fulfillment cannot be scaled by anyone who lacks control of body, mind, and emotions.

Discipline, to me, means the ability to carry out a resolution long
after the mood and enthusiasm has left you. It also means doing what
you say you're going to do.

Discipline brings freedom and peace to your life. A disciplined
person is not at the whim or mercy of external circumstances, but is
in control of what he thinks, feels, says, and does. An undisciplined
person is lazy, undirected, and usually unhappy. Discipline of the mind
leads to discipline of the body. And from a disciplined body comes an
exhilarated mind.

We cannot discipline ourselves with the larger things of life until we understand that discipline must be achieved with the smaller things. It's been my experience that through discipline in small things, greater tasks that once seemed difficult become easier. For example, it takes discipline to sit at my desk each day to write this book. As the days go by, however, the writing becomes more enjoyable and I see my vision of a book come into fruition. Similarly, it takes discipline to eat healthy foods all the time and to exercise regularly. But if I take on this adventure of healthy living one day at a time, I will reach the thirtieth day without feeling overwhelmed by the scope of the task.

We can't address the topic of discipline without also venturing into the power of conditioning. The way we have been conditioned to behave affects all areas of our lives.

How often do you eat compulsively rather than from true hunger? Think of your eating behavior at social gatherings, at the movies, or when you're watching television or attending sports events. Discipline yourself to eat slowly and only when you're truly hungry.

When I've been out skiing, I sometimes notice a small ball of snow that begins to roll down from the top of the mountain. At that point, the snow is easy to stop. But if the ball continues to roll, it may grow steadily bigger until an immense mass of several tons descends. At that size, it is impossible to stop. Our desires work the same way. They gain power and strength through repetition. Repetition is the key to mastery, or to failure. When a negative desire first surfaces, we must eradicate it quickly and firmly. When you have a desire to eat junk food, don't give in. Exercise discipline. Choose something healthy to eat or abstain from snacking at that time.

When you repeat negative behavior, it develops into a bad habit. To eradicate your negative conditioning, make a twenty-one-day agreement with yourself. It takes twenty-one days to form a new habit or break an old one. Let's say that at mealtime you want to stop eating before you feel stuffed. Make an agreement with yourself to do that. Resolve to stick with your agreement every day for twenty-one days. If you skip a day, you must begin the cycle again. By the twenty-first day, your mind and body will stop resisting the change you're trying to make. Three weeks isn't a long time. If you find your mind coming up with excuses, as it will, you can maintain discipline by reminding yourself that you only have to continue for twenty-one days.

I have been incorporating this tip into my life for thirty-five years. On the first of each month, I make an agreement with myself to give up some unhealthful habit or to reinforce a positive pattern. In this way, I make twelve beneficial changes in my life each year.

In my book *Health Bliss*, which is part of a 3-book Blissful Living set, you will find a two-page chart for the 21-day program that you can copy and use monthly. There is also a one-page 21-Day Agreement form available at *www.SusanSmithJones.com*.

Honoring your agreements with yourself boosts your self-esteem. When I don't do this, I feel lousy. But when I stay disciplined and do what I say I'm going to do, I feel empowered. I have great respect for people who keep their word. And I lose respect for those who don't.

One of my favorite heroes was John Wooden, basketball coach for UCLA. For twenty-seven years, he molded champions on and off the court. His leadership generated excitement all over campus and touched the lives of millions around the country. His unparalleled string of victories and National Collegiate Athletic Association championships remain the benchmark for basketball teams everywhere. One of the main ingredients in what Wooden called the "pyramid of success" is practicing discipline in every aspect of life and keeping one's word with oneself. (Coach Wooden graciously wrote the foreword for my book *Be Healthy~Stay Balanced*.)

One way to begin to master this art of discipline and to see immediate results is to schedule time every morning to meditate. Even if you are not yet a committed disciple on the spiritual path, meditate for the practical health benefits. I have discovered that by being disciplined with my meditation, I have more discipline in other areas of my life. What's more, being disciplined brings me more peace. And it's from a more peaceful mind and heart that I am consequently able to welcome more discipline in other aspects of my life.

Now is the time to become a disciplined person. Enrich every aspect of your life with self-discipline. You will discover, as I have, that discipline is the road to freedom, mastery, and peace.

Choose to be self-disciplined today.

~

It is neither wealth nor splendor, but tranquility and occupation which give happiness.

—THOMAS JEFFERSON

Good habits are your best helpers; preserve their force by stimulating them with good actions. Bad habits are your worst enemies, against your will they make you do the things that hurt you most. They are detrimental to your physical, social, mental, moral, and spiritual happiness. Stave bad habits by refusing to give them any further food of bad actions.

—PARAMAHANSA YOGANANDA

Today's Affirmation & Action Step

I make discipline a way of life for myself. My mind is disciplined, which means my body is disciplined. Thank you, Spirit of Life within me, for letting your discipline shine through in everything I think, feel, say, and do.

Whatever you say you are going to do today, do it. Keep your word with yourself and others. Also, make a special agreement with yourself to get something done about which you have been procrastinating. No excuses today. Get it done. Think self-discipline today.

Day 15

Cultivate the Joy of Ritual and Ceremony

It had done me good to be somewhat parched by the heat and drenched by the rain of life.

—HENRY WADSWORTH LONGFELLOW

Every human being has a great . . . gift to care, to be compassionate, to be present to the other, to listen, to hear, and to receive.

—HENRI NOUWEN

Our planet, Mother Earth, is alive, radiant and calling us back home. Too often we forget our connection to the earth and we create a separation between it and us. Earth and its atmosphere provide such constant and reliable support that we take them for granted and thus unconsciously abuse them.

The American Indians are known for their connection with the earth, and I believe we have much to learn from them. It's time for all of us to reawaken to the life force that connects us to Mother Earth. Through ritual and ceremony, we can touch the sacredness within ourselves and within the earth. We are divine beings, thus sacred; the planet is a divine entity, thus sacred. We are united by a holy umbilical cord. Wherever we walk is holy ground: the earth empowers us. We can and must respect and acknowledge her presence. By joining energies, we can become whole again.

You can go to a place of natural power on this planet and, with ritual and ceremony, feel transformed and renewed. Or you can bring the same experience to your daily activities. This is what I would like to concentrate on in this chapter—bringing sacredness into your life through everyday activities and natural occurrences. For more detailed information on this topic, please refer to my book *The Joy Factor*.

Ritual is the act of taking something ordinary and raising it to the level of the extraordinary. It's taking a daily occurrence and empowering yourself by performing this activity with higher consciousness and awareness. Rituals help us gain perspective on changes, offer tradition, support a greater sense of balance, and help us relate to one another. If you want to recognize life's changes consciously or bring greater meaning and understanding to the customs you already practice, I highly recommend incorporating ritual into your life. In earlier chapters, I've mentioned the healing power of food. Preparing a meal in a loving way can become a ritual of self-care. You not only gain nutrients, but also the deeper sense of connecting with nature's elements.

I am passionate about connecting with Mother Earth and including special rituals in my life. For years, I've been striving to live from the highest and most sacred parts of myself. One of the things I love to do alone or with close friends is to hike in the Santa Monica Mountains. Sometimes I hike briskly from beginning to end just to get an aerobic workout. Other times my hike becomes a ritual, a sacred adventure with Mother Nature. During a recent ritual hike with a close friend, we talked about what we hoped to gain, to learn, to focus on during the hike as well as your lives in general. We hiked with attention to the beauty of nature around us. During the hike, we came to a waterfall and sprinkled water on our heads, each of us feeling empowered in our own personal way. I experienced this water ceremony as a sort of baptism, purifying me and washing away all blockages to the awareness of God's presence. By the end of the hike, it felt like I was *walking on air*.

You can make anything personally sacred for yourself. Maybe one particular hike is a ritual for claiming prosperity and abundance as you pay attention to nature's abundance all around you. Another day, the ritual hike might be needed in order to open you up to healing and greater health.

I've grown to see every time I'm out in nature as an opportunity for ritual, to remember who I am and my connection with Mother Earth. I always remember to include ritual and ceremony when there is a new moon or a full moon, at the start of the four seasonal changes, even at sunsets and sunrises. Sometimes I perform these rituals alone, sometimes with a close friend, and every so often in a small group or workshop setting somewhere in the world.

You can create your own special ritual outside of the 30-day program offered in this book. For example, pick a period of 10–40 days. On the first day, write down everything you want to surrender to God, which might be everything in your life. It took me about two hours to write everything down the last time I did this. I wrote about my dreams and goals, my friends and family, my health and body, my career, and all my fears. After reading over the pages, I wrote out a declaration that for ___ days I would: turn everything in my life over to God and my angels; pray and meditate; eat only healthy, colorful, organic foods; and, to the best of my ability, live in the presence of love and focus on the things I was grateful for. My goal was to live more as a spiritual being than a human being. I would experience not my will, but God's will in my life. I then signed this paper, folded it up, and placed it on my meditation altar, where I sit daily in quiet reflection and prayer.

The following morning, Day 1 of my program, I went down to the beach alone and walked barefoot by the water, talking to God and my guardian angels. I was aware of my connection with Mother Earth and could feel her energy and strength. After the walk, I meditated and then waded into the water. With my hands cupped, I poured water over my head and body to cleanse my body and mind. I then went back to the sand and let the healing sun dry me off. Could I have begun the program without a ritual? Of course. But I wanted to set a tone and to empower myself. Ritual gives my life richness, fullness, and sacredness.

The moon lends herself to rituals, too. Traditionally, all over the planet, people mark the phases of the moon on their calendars each month. A new moon occurs every twenty-eight days. Traditionally, this was a time for planting seeds. On a metaphysical level, this time of the month is good for planting the seeds of change we want to manifest in our lives. According to the universal law of cause and effect, if we create change in ourselves, changes will manifest around us.

By incorporating ritual and ceremony, you can add dimension and sacredness to any ordinary activity. When you view your body and life as sacred, life becomes richer. You feel and connect with Mother Earth in a deeper bond of respect, honor, and love. Sacredness becomes a way of life. Through the work of some of the world's finest photographers, the magic that surrounds sacred sites, places of power, and natural shrines is evoked and preserved. Writing by contemporary thinkers and by authors of the past opens a variety of possibilities for relating to the earth. This book can serve as a doorway into a place of new awareness within you for Mother Earth.

Cultivate the joy of ritual and ceremony.

~

So to yield to life is to solve the unsolvable.

—LAO-TZU

It is one of the most beautiful compensations of this life that no man can sincerely try to help another without helping himself.

—RALPH WALDO EMERSON

Today's Affirmation & Action Step

I am grateful for all Mother Earth has given me. Her abundance and beauty are everywhere. In stillness, I listen for her guidance and know that every step I take is on holy ground. Divine love, flowing through us both, connects our hearts.

Bring ritual into your day. Perhaps sit down to a cup of tea and let each moment of drinking the tea be sacred to you. Tea is a hug in a cup to me. Or honor this day and Mother Earth by adding a new plant to your garden or home. Today, think about creating sacred ritual.

Day 16

Celebrate the Miracle of Your Body with Exercise

I still get wildly enthusiastic about little things . . . I play with leaves. I skip down the street, and run against the wind.

—LEO BUSCAGLIA

Far away there in the sunshine are my highest aspirations. I may not reach them, but I can look at them to see their beauty, believe in them, and try to follow where they lead.

—LOUISA MAY ALCOTT

Modern living has channeled the average American into an increasingly sedentary existence. We human beings, however, were designed and built for movement, and our bodies have not adapted well to this reduced level of activity. As we've learned, what we put into our bodies is of utmost importance, but how we use our bodies is just as integral.

For many adults with sedentary occupations, physical activity provides an outlet for job-related tensions or mental fatigue. In addition, exercise can boost spirits and help us feel good about ourselves. Exercise also aids in weight control or reduction, improves posture, and increases energy. Further, proper exercise can often prevent or correct lower back pain. In fact, about half of the cases of lower back pain I've seen can be traced to poor muscle tone and to inflexibility.

Research also indicates that much of the degeneration of bodily function and structure associated with premature aging seems to be reduced by a program of vigorous, regular exercise.

Regular exercise is necessary to develop and maintain not only an optimal level of health, but also a youthful appearance, mental clarity, and high energy. Regular exercise increases muscle strength and endurance. It enhances the function of the lungs, heart, and blood vessels; it increases the flexibility of the joints; and improves coordination and efficiency of movement.

Today, we will concentrate on how exercise contributes to our self-image, happiness, and peace of mind. "A sound mind in a sound body" is a traditional British motto. Researchers are finding, however, that there's much more to the adage than might first appear. It seems that our sense of happiness and well-being depends on how much exercise we get. Dr. Malcolm Carruthers believes that "most people could ban the blues with a simple, vigorous ten-minute exercise session three times a week." He came to this conclusion after spending four years studying the effect of norepinephrine on two hundred people. Norepinephrine is a depression-destroying hormone, "the chemical key to happiness," according to Carruthers. Ten minutes of exercise doubles the level of norepinephrine in the body.

Enkephalin is another spirit-lifting chemical produced in the brain during vigorous aerobic exercise. It is responsible for the feeling known as runner's high. Enkephalin is a type of endorphin, a morphine-like chemical that serves as a natural opiate, increasing pain tolerance and producing euphoric feelings. A study at Massachusetts General Hospital found a rise of more than 145 percent in endorphins during one hour of vigorous exercise. So you might want to heed the words of Paul Dudley White, MD, who once said: "Walk your dog every day, whether you have a dog or not."

Exercise can work in conjunction with psychotherapy to alleviate depression, according to work done at the Menninger Clinic in Topeka, Kansas. "It's not a panacea, but it is a useful adjunct for treating depression," says the clinic's Robert Conroy. One of Conroy's hypotheses is that exercise boosts self-image by changing an individual's worldview from that of passive bystander to active participant. People who exercise believe they have control over their health and the quality of their lives.

Exercise also releases tension, which helps alleviate tension-related bodily malfunctions such as ulcers, migraine headaches, asthma, skin eruptions, high blood pressure, and heart disease. And exercise also leads to a good night's sleep, a key to mental well-being.

Aerobic activity—vigorous, rhythmical activities such as jogging, brisk walking, running, swimming, aerobic dancing, rowing, cross-country skiing, hiking, cycling, and stair-climbing—is the kind of exercise that produces truly beneficial psychological and biochemical changes. It appears to send messages to the brain as well as the endocrine system to shape up and feel good.

Exercise is a rewarding and enjoyable means of taking control of your psychological and physical well-being. A well-designed physical fitness program can add years of fulfillment, vibrant health, and peace of mind to your life. (And that knowledge alone has a potent positive effect on mental well-being.)

Celebrate the miracle of your body with exercise.

∽

Continuous effort—not strength or intelligence—is the key to unlocking our potential.

—Winston Churchill

Shake yourself awake. Develop a hobby. Let the winds of enthusiasm sweep through you. Live today with gusto.

—Dale Carnegie

Today's Affirmation & Action Step

I love to exercise, and I do so regularly. Exercise brings me more energy, mental clarity, self-confidence, and peace of mind. Taking care of my body is my way of saying thank you to Spirit for my health and my life.

Find a way to exercise today. Take a walk, go to the gym, or simply step in place while watching TV. Be active today. Think about how much you want to get into peak shape.

Day 17

Choose to Use Age-Defying Natural Remedies

Each patient carries his own doctor inside him.

—ALBERT SCHWEITZER

When you put your force and energy behind something, the results will be powerful.

—ALEXANDRA STODDARD

If we were to trace the roots of modern medicine, they would lead us to the rich soil of Earth's fields and forests. For centuries, native cultures have used indigenous plants in their healing practices. Over 4,500 years ago, Chinese and Indian healers began to organize bodies of knowledge about the medicinal properties of herbs. In the first century AD, the Greek physician Dioscorides compiled a guide to five hundred healing herbs, which endured as the standard text of medical arts through the Middle Ages. The European desire for curative herbs and spices of the Far East motivated Columbus to set sail in the fifteenth century so that he could find a shortcut to these lands. When he encountered the New World, he stumbled upon the herbal riches of North America and the vast knowledge of healing practices passed down from the Mayan, Aztec, and other native civilizations.

Humans used to rely almost entirely upon plants to treat illnesses both minor and serious until only about fifty years ago. It wasn't until scientists discovered how to make purified and concentrated derivatives of plants that modern pharmaceuticals rose to prominence. In the American health-care system today, whole plants are rarely used therapeutically, but eighty of 150 of the most popular pharmaceutical products sold contain active ingredients derived from herbal sources, including morphine (derived from opium poppy), cough-relieving ephedrine (from *Ephedra sinica*), and digoxin, also known as digitalis, which treats congestive heart failure (derived from the common foxglove).

Yet despite modern medicine's debt to nature's pharmacy, traditional herbal medicine and Western (allopathic) medicine took divergent paths in the twentieth century. Synthesized drugs began to take priority over the original botanical sources. American medical universities excluded herbal healing modalities from their curricula because such practices were regarded to be based in superstition rather than science. In India, under British rule, the herbal traditions of Ayurvedic medicine were pushed aside in favor of Western methods.

Today, herbal and allopathic medicines' paths are crossing once again. The dangerous side effects of some pharmaceuticals, as evidenced in the recall of drugs such as thalidomide and Fen-Phen, have alerted the medical community to the potential risks of chemically synthesized substances. And a new understanding of the role of diet, stress, and lifestyle in the development of diseases has prompted a renewed appreciation for natural interventions. Perhaps most important, a growing body of scientific literature is revealing that much of the wisdom of the ancients was scientifically sound; specific herbs and foods can indeed have a positive impact on essential physiological functions and help protect us from disease.

In seeking remedies from the farm, not the pharmacy, we reconnect with the natural environment and with the traditions of our ancestors. As I mentioned in the introduction, my grandmother Fritzie taught me how to take care of my body using only natural remedies. She taught me how to use foods, herbs, and spices as well as other lifestyle choices to support healthy digestion, elimination, and sleep; restore weakened immunity; calm stress; soothe colds and flu; keep my heart healthy and bones strong; and promote detoxification and rejuvenation. Because of her wisdom, I have never in my life had to take medication. My grandmother followed Native American wisdom, which says, "When you need an answer, listen to Nature."

Across America, we are seeing a rebirth of natural healing, as natural remedies begin to play a more visible role in mainstream health care today. The overuse of antibiotics in recent decades has created deadly antibiotic-resistant bacteria. Throughout the world, there is growing concern that many illness-causing microorganisms such as bacteria, viruses, fungi, and parasites are becoming resistant to the drugs used to fight them. Prevention of illness is the key, but when one does get sick, understanding how to use natural remedies that have been proven over centuries to heal our bodies can be very helpful, and they generally don't have many of the harmful side effects that pharmaceuticals can.

In my travels and studies over four decades, I have witnessed tremendous results in myself, my family and friends, and my clients through using nature's plants as medicine. Although you always want to consult your physician, especially if you are taking any type of allopathic medicine, the following is just a brief sampling of some natural remedies that really work. For more information, please refer to my website *www.SusanSmithJones. com* and click on Natural Remedies and *Renew Your Life*.

Before I present twelve of my favorite age-defying superfoods, I want to first define what a superfood (or, as I coined it more than thirty years ago, a *naturefood*) is. All foods are not equal. Some are full of calories and void of nutrition, while others are low on calories and so packed with nutrition that they earn the title of superfood. There's a difference between food volume versus nutritional potency: you don't need a lot of food to get a lot of nutrition. For example, blueberries are considered a superfood because they contain significant amounts of antioxidants, anthocyanins, vitamin C, manganese, and dietary fiber with relatively few calories. Superfoods are the best whole foods out there, but no one is a magic bullet; make sure you include many different superfoods in your diet to help maintain optimal health.

Eat Your Way to Vibrant Health

On this seventeenth day of your new healthy lifestyle, get off to a great start with any one of these twelve age-defying, plant-based foods that also happen to be heart-strengthening, cancer-busting, energy-boosting, detox-enhancing, and body-slimming superfoods. They are all easy to find in your supermarket or natural foods store.

Almonds: Two ounces of almonds give you more than 50 percent of your daily requirement of magnesium, a mineral that's important for heart health. Eating almonds every day for at least a month has been shown to reduce cholesterol and lower other risk factors for heart disease. A study also suggests that almonds may reduce the risk of colon cancer. Sprinkle them in salads or grind into a pastry.

Apples: Eating an apple a day could very well keep the cardiologist away. Current studies suggest that eating apples regularly reduces the risk of stroke and heart attack. They lower cholesterol and also appear to decrease the risk of lung cancer. Eating them whole, with the skin on, provides the highest level of nutritional value.

Avocados: Avocados have more protein than any other fruit. Sometimes known as nature's butter, they have only about a quarter of the fat calories contained in the same weight of dairy butter. Ounce for ounce, they also provide more heart-healthy monounsaturated fat, vitamin E, folate, potassium, and fiber than other fruits. You can mash an avocado onto whole grain bread and into baked potatoes, and even use it as a hydrating mask. Avocados also exceed other fruits as a source of the powerful antioxidant lutein, which appears to protect arteries from hardening and the eyes from cataracts and macular degeneration.

Bananas: Monkeys' favorite food is among the most nutritious of tropical fruits. Fiber from green, unripe bananas reduces bad cholesterol and increases good cholesterol by as much as 30 percent, while a ripe banana is one of the best ways to soothe an upset stomach. Bananas are a wonderful source of energy, can relieve heartburn, and also help decrease the risk of stroke. Besides perhaps strawberries, no other fresh fruit is higher in minerals.

Broccoli: Broccoli has more than twice as much protein as steak—11.2 grams per 100 calories compared with only 5.4 grams. (Most of the calories in meat come from fat, but the calories in green veggies come from protein.) Broccoli is one of nature's most potent superfoods. It has proven effective against cancer, heart disease, and a host of other serious conditions. Its powerful sulforaphane content delivers a double punch to cancer-causing chemicals, destroying any carcinogenic compounds that you have ingested, then creating enzymes that eat up any carcinogens left over from that reaction. It also contains indole-3-carbinol, which helps your body metabolize estrogen, potentially warding off breast cancer.

Cinnamon: This ancient and versatile spice (obtained from the bark of Asian evergreens) helps to relieve bloating and stabilize blood sugar. Cinnamon contains methylhydroxychalcone polymer (MHCP), which speeds up the processing of sugar in your body. So putting cinnamon sticks in your tea or water, or sprinkling just a tiny amount on desserts, fruits, and cereal, and into smoothies, will make your insulin release much more efficient, which may slow aging and help ward off diabetes and obesity. (I purchase my cinnamon sticks and all of my spices and herbs at *www.PennHerb.com*.)

Garlic: Herbalists have used garlic to treat all sorts of diseases for thousands of years. As well as being scrumptious, garlic is a rich source of the sulphur compounds that keep your body chemistry in balance, fighting infections, slowing down the production of cholesterol, and lowering blood pressure. There is even evidence that garlic helps to fight cancer and improves the action of the liver and the gallbladder. Add garlic to your cooking and salad dressings, or roast unpeeled cloves for forty to forty-five minutes, then peel and mash them into purées and sauces. I also recommend adding the nutritional supplement Kyolic Aged Garlic Extract to your diet. Call 1-800-421-2998 for a free sample of Kyolic or other Wakunaga of America products. (For more information, visit *www.Kyolic.com*, as well as my website.)

Oats: Inexpensive, readily available, and incredibly easy to incorporate into your life, oats contain twice as much protein as brown rice and are an excellent source of complex carbohydrates to maintain your energy levels throughout the day. They improve your resistance to stress, help regulate the thyroid, soothe the nervous and digestive systems, reduce cigarette cravings, and stabilize blood sugar levels.

Parsley: This common herb is a powerhouse of nutrients that rejuvenate and detoxify. Include it when you make fresh juice. Nibble a few leaves when you want your breath to be sweeter. Chop it into salads, soups, sandwiches, and pasta dishes. Parsley is also a stress-buster, and studies have shown it to be effective in reducing depression, lowering cholesterol, and strengthening kidneys. Many herbalists recommend parsley to relieve the symptoms of rheumatism and PMS.

Parsnips: Parsnips could be nicknamed the "beauty food" because of the way their nutritional components help strengthen hair and nails and improve skin quality. People who suffer from acne or skin disorders will appreciate the skin-flattering benefits of the parsnip's unique balance of potassium, phosphorus, and vitamin C.

Pomegranates: This dark-red fruit is hot news these days—especially as a juice. Pomegranates are packed full of disease-fighting antioxidants. Some studies suggest that they offer almost three times more antioxidants than other popular sources such as green tea, red wine, blueberry juice, and cranberry juice. They also contain potassium, fiber, vitamin C, and niacin, all of which contribute to increased energy and good health. Pomegranates have also been shown to reduce plaque buildup in arteries by up to 44 percent.

Tomatoes: This beautiful low-calorie fruit is jam-packed with nutrients and phytochemicals, which boost the body's immune defenses. Whether in soups, sauces, or salads, tomatoes are rich in vitamins B and C and also contain lycopene, which appears to act as a protective factor against cancer (and may also benefit the heart). Cooked tomatoes contain more lycopene than raw, and most of the nutritional value is contained in the skin, so, ounce for ounce, cherry tomatoes are more nutritious than large ones.

Please refer to my full-color recipe book, *Recipes for Health Bliss*, which includes more than 150 color photographs and 250 delicious, easy-to-prepare, and nutritious recipes. As a culinary instructor for over twenty-five years, I have included my best-of-the-best recipes in this book that your entire family will love. There are also more scrumptious recipes in my books *Health Bliss, Be Healthy~Stay Balanced,* and *The Healing Power of NatureFoods,* as well as on my website *www.SusanSmithJones.com.*

Choose to use age-defying natural remedies.

~

Everything lives, everything is animated, everything seems to speak to me of my passion, everything invites me to cherish it.

—ANNE DE LENCLOS

You can accomplish anything if you do not accept limitations. . . . Whatever you make up your mind to do, you can do.

—PARAMAHANSA YOGANANDA

Today's Affirmation & Action Step

I select from a rainbow of natural foods. Whether breakfast, lunch, dinner, or a snack, I enjoy eating foods grown close to nature. I am grateful for the abundance of energy and vitality I feel as a result. I love my body and take care of it each day with healthy foods and positive thoughts.

Select a natural, colorful fruit or veggie that is out of the ordinary for you and eat it today. Eat slowly and savor every bite. Imagine the energy of the food infusing your body with vitality. Think colorful produce today.

Day 18

Cultivate an Attitude of Gratitude and Humility

The mind of man is capable of anything because everything is in it—all of the past, as well as all of the future.

—JOSEPH CONRAD

Let us be grateful to people who make us happy; they are the charming gardeners who make our souls blossom.

—MARCEL PROUST

An attitude of gratitude opens our consciousness to all the blessings God has showered on us. It's like a magnet that attracts good and multiplies joy and happiness. Just as all good things proceed from a peaceful mind, so all things are nourished from a grateful heart.

In 1789, President George Washington introduced the first national day of Thanksgiving and prayer to be devoted "to the services of that great and glorious Being who is the beneficent author of all the good that was, that is, and that will be; that we may then all unite in rendering unto Him our sincere and humble thanks. . . ." During the presidency of Abraham Lincoln, Thanksgiving Day became an official national holiday. Two of our wisest presidents thus acknowledged our need to remember our dependency on the goodness of God and the need for peacefulness.

Sometimes in life we give thanks only when things seem to be going well. When things go badly, we lose sight of all our blessings. The Greek philosopher Epicurus warned us, "Do not spoil what you have by desiring what you have not." Praise everything in your life—even the things that may not look like blessings. *Your soul becomes more refined and receptive to good when you live from a grateful heart.* Gratitude and thanksgiving are qualities too often misunderstood or not exercised. Gratitude is a dynamic energy that allows you to exert a mighty influence on your world. It is like a connecting bridge that links you to all possible channels of good in your life. Giving thanks multiplies what you have. It increases abundance. Jesus did it. Elijah did it. This same power is within you.

I have a friend whose income barely covers her bills each month. And every month, she complains and gets depressed about her insufficient income. After a couple of months of hearing her complaining, I said to her that she could begin to change her financial situation by changing her attitude from lack and limitation to one of thanksgiving. So I told her that for one month, she was to think only grateful thoughts about her work, income, bills, and abundance. When the bills came in, I suggested she bless each one, giving thanks for the service and product provided. I encouraged her to write, "Thank you, with love," on each check. She admitted to me that she found this quite difficult to do the first month. But within two months, not only did her attitude change about paying bills, but she also actually had some money left over. Abundance began coming to her from sources expected and unexpected. When she opened up the channels and acknowledged God as her source, her blessings began to multiply.

By appreciating what we have, we increase our ability to harvest the abundance of God's blessings. Every day, think about all you have to be grateful for. It's a perfect way to start each morning after your time of prayer and meditation. Throughout the day, continue your praise and thanksgiving. For example, I give thanks for things like healthy foods, the beautiful clouds, pure water after a lengthy and vigorous workout, the friends in my life, and the comfort of my bed after a long day's work. Even when I'm facing a challenge or am having difficulty with someone, I give thanks for that, too, knowing God will provide the answer and I will learn from the circumstance.

Humility is a quality of the heart. It's having or showing a modest estimate of one's own importance. It's also believing in something bigger than you. For me, humility comes from realizing that Spirit makes all things possible.

When you know that you are one with the all-loving heart-light inside you, and it's not you but the Divine Mind through you that accomplishes the good, then everything is in better perspective. You're able to see how your ego tries to battle for recognition and esteem. True humility is not a weakness. It is to be ever aware that we live in the heart of Love and to affirm, "Not my will, but Thy will be done." If we feel this in our hearts, then we can let go of our personal desires and the frustration of their nonfulfillment, remaining content in the greater desire to do whatever God wants us to do. This is true humility: to put God uppermost in our lives.

Cultivate an attitude of gratitude and humility today.

~

Every day should be a day of thanksgiving for the gifts of life: sunshine, water, and the luscious fruits and greens that are indirect gifts of the Great Giver.

—Paramahansa Yogananda

Today's Affirmation & Action Steps

Today I sing a song of praise and gratitude. I see each person in my life as God's gift to me. In each encounter of this day I learn, grow, and deepen in my awareness of Love's wonder and blessing. I dedicate my life to doing God's will and to creating my best life.

Sometime before you go to bed tonight, write down at least ten things for which you are grateful. If you can write more, go for it! Write as many as you can and feel the joy and thanksgiving you have for each blessing on your list. Think gratitude today.

Day 19

Celebrate a Serene and Balanced Existence

Dreams are the touchstones of our character.

—HENRY DAVID THOREAU

The skies can't keep their secret! They tell it to the hills—the hills just tell the orchards—and they the daffodils.

—EMILY DICKINSON

People are in such a rush these days—talking fast, eating fast, moving fast. Given our current pace, we barely have time to relax and cultivate relationships with our spouses and children, friends and nature, much less with God. Is it any wonder that stress-related diseases are on the rise?

I see this as a sickness of epidemic proportions—a busy-ness or hurry sickness. Here are some of the signs of hurry sickness. See if you identify with any of them:

1. Erratic Driving Pattern—You routinely drive fast and run yellow lights, you jockey for position and constantly change lanes, and you're impatient with other drivers.

2. Hurried Eating Habits—You eat in a rush, often while on the go.

3. Rushed Communication Style—You talk fast, have problems communicating how you feel, and rarely find the time to give emotional support to your family and friends.

4. Lack of Family Involvement—You are not home much and when you are, you're tired and tend to withdraw, or you sit in front of the TV.

5. Limited Leisure Activities—Your hurried life is so full of undone chores and responsibilities that relaxing has become even more difficult, if not impossible; vacations are rare; when you're not doing something productive, you experience anxiety and guilt.

We all want to live in a way that allows us to emerge as winners. The trick is to enjoy the process along the way, as I communicate in my book *The Joy Factor* and throughout my program *Renew Your Life*.

Oftentimes the cause for our hurriedness is economic—we must make more money to pay for our chosen lifestyles. Sometimes the cause lies in simply having too much to do or feeling that something is wrong if we aren't busy. But beyond these reasons is something deeper—a lifestyle that leaves certain basic needs unfulfilled. By crowding our schedules with more—more socializing, more eating, more work, more activity, and more appointments—we are trying to fill the emptiness within.

When you direct your attention and your energies outward, you lose sense of the wonder, beauty, and magnificence within you, from which true happiness, joy, and peace originate. By slowing down and redirecting your energies inward, you can train your brain to relax and you can ultimately change your life.

One of the world's leading experts on the brain is Herbert Benson, MD, author of *The Relaxation Response*. He developed what he calls the "relaxation response"—the body's ability to enter into a scientifically definable state characterized by an overall reduction of its metabolic rate, with lowered blood pressure, decreased rate of breathing, slower brain waves, and a lowered heart rate. According to Benson, this state of relaxation also acts as a door to a renewed mind and a changed life, a feeling of wholeness and, often, expanded awareness. Physiological changes occur when you are relaxed; there is increased communication between the two sides of the brain, resulting in feelings variously described as well-being, unboundedness, harmony, infinite connection, and peak experience.

To reach this level of calmness, there are several things you can do. One approach is to relax your body progressively, beginning with your toes and ending with your head. For example, you might breathe slowly and deeply as you say to yourself, "My toes are relaxed, my feet are relaxed, my back is relaxed," and on until you've covered your entire body. Then rest for a while in the quiet and silence. Another way to relax is to visualize yourself feeling relaxed and peaceful. Use your imagination. You can also listen to the audio programs available on my website, especially the ones titled *Celebrate Life!* and *Wired to Meditate.*

One of my favorite ways to relax wherever I am is to visit my inner sanctuary. I do this several times a week, for just a few minutes, and I always come back more relaxed and peaceful. You can create a sanctuary within yourself where you can go anytime just by closing your eyes and desiring to be there. Your sanctuary is an ideal place of mental relaxation, tranquility, beauty, safety, and calmness.

Something else you can do at work or at home to relax your mind and body is to look at a picture of a beautiful landscape. In my home, I have a couple posters I purchased from the Sierra Club that depict scenes from nature. Whenever I look at them, I can sense a difference in how I feel.

Another approach to relaxation and calmness comes from simply breathing. Take a few minutes and breathe slowly and deeply, really focusing on your breath. You will find that this calms and soothes you and helps you to slow down and get centered.

You might recite your favorite inspirational quote, passage, or affirmation a few times, slowly and deliberately, while giving it your total attention. One of my favorite affirmations is "This day I choose to spend in perfect peace." I also use "I am the ever-renewing, ever-unfolding radiant expression of infinite life, health, wealth, joy and wisdom, unconditional love, and universal peace."

When you make an effort to relax, don't feel that you must live your life in slow motion. Not at all. You can maintain activity. Your goal is to touch your inner fountain of calmness and bring that calmness to everything you do. Being calm brings clarity, richness, and divinity to your life. Even in your activity, you will be aware of Love's presence.

I know of no more effective way of bringing about relaxation, calmness, and a slower pace than to meditate regularly. All of the physiological changes described in Benson's book occur during meditation. The calmness you feel during your daily practice will stay with you in everything you do. You'll find that your life will become more rewarding, you'll accomplish more, you'll have more fun, and you won't have to miss out on celebrating life. (Please refer to Day 29 for more information on meditation.)

Celebrate a serene and balanced existence.

∾

I wish you all the joy that you can wish.

—WILLIAM SHAKESPEARE

Always dream and shoot higher than you know you can do.

—WILLIAM FAULKNER

Today's Affirmation & Action Step

I choose to live with balance and plan my days so that I am relaxed and serene. I live by my own time schedule, not the time schedule of the world and everyone around me. Each morning, I enjoy a peaceful start to my day. I start and end my days on a relaxed, positive note.

Participate in the progressive relaxation I described in this chapter. Either sitting or lying, relax your body from your toes up to your head as you breathe deeply. Focus on each body part as you relax and think of nothing else. Think peaceful relaxation today.

Day 20

Choose to Be Prosperous and to Attract Abundance

One can live magnificently in the world, if one knows how to work and how to love.

—LEO TOLSTOY

If you look at what you have in life, you'll always have more. If you look at what you don't have, you'll never have enough.

—OPRAH WINFREY

For many people, abundance and prosperity are tied to their level of self-esteem. You make a good living, pay your bills, and save money, so you feel successful. I define success in a different light. Success is not a matter of how much money you have, how many possessions you've collected, or what type of lifestyle you choose to live; success can be measured only by the degree to which you have inner peace and, no matter the circumstance or situation, can remain peaceful, calm, and happy. One of my favorite passages in the Bible (Matt. 6:33) is: "Seek first His kingdom and his righteousness, and all these things will be given to you as well."

I know what some of you might be thinking. Being peaceful doesn't pay my bills or put food on the table. But that's where you may be mistaken. Abundance and prosperity begin inside you. Believe me when I say I speak from experience.

Many years ago, it seemed that no matter what I did or what I'd accomplished, I continued to feel lack and limitation in my life. When money finally came to me, it disappeared almost instantly. I was frustrated, depressed, and confused. One day I decided to do everything possible to change the situation and to live the life God created for me. I read books, attended prosperity lectures and workshops, prayed and meditated, and after a while, I finally put all the pieces of the puzzle together.

First, it's important to realize that your thoughts and beliefs affect your level of abundance. Do you feel worthy of abundance? Do you wish for abundance and at the same time worry about how you'll pay your bills? Do you even believe that there's enough money to go around? You will attract to yourself what you believe to be true. Have your beliefs and thoughts closed the doors to prosperity?

For me, choosing to open the doors to prosperity also involved being aware of all the abundance around me. Just look at nature—the oceans, the clouds, the sky, the mountains and rivers, the stars; there couldn't be a better lesson in abundance. I asked myself, "From where does all this come?" God is the source of this supply of abundance. When I acted from this awareness, my level of prosperity changed.

You see, up until that point, I had been looking outside myself for the source of my supply. It's not outside you. It's within you. *Everything you need to be happy, to be prosperous, and to live abundantly, is inside you right now.* When you love the Divine with all of your being, you draw His kingdom into your consciousness, and His abundance is made evident in your world. You must know that and *feel* it. If you think in terms of scarcity, you will manifest limitation. Similarly, if you think thoughts of abundance, you will manifest sufficiency, success, and happiness. *All the fortune is in the follow-up and follow-through.*

To open the floodgates of abundance, you must begin by giving away what you have. Some call this tithing; some call it sharing. Paramahansa Yogananda wrote in *Where There Is Light,* "Unselfishness is the governing principle in the law of prosperity." When you give of yourself to another person or group, you always receive more than you give. We are all one, so to give to another is to give to yourself. But keep in mind that your giving must always be guided by Spirit and not stem from guilt. My financial situation turned around quickly when I started tithing and giving to others. I always receive my gifts back, multiplied.

I realize that it might feel scary to give when you think you can barely pay your bills. Start with small donations and gifts, always blessing the money and being grateful that you are able to share what you have. Remember the wise words of Lao-Tzu: "A journey of a thousand miles must first begin with a single step."

Next, it's important to love what you do. Do you feel passion and enthusiasm for your work? Do you get up every morning eager to get started? Or do you dread how you spend your day? A recent national poll revealed that 95 percent of people working in America do not enjoy what they do! This is a staggering statistic. For years, I have done extensive research on people who are successful, and I have been a life coach for many of them. It's clear to me that achievements and financial rewards are directly related to the enjoyment we derive from our work and the service we provide to our communities and the world.

Right livelihood is predicated upon a conscious choice. Yet, too often, we live our lives according to what others value. When you consciously choose to enter into your work, you can participate fully and know you are making a difference. Sometimes this takes courage and perseverance, but your life will be enriched.

I have a friend who went into dental school right after college because his parents had always wanted him to be a dentist. Although dentistry wasn't his calling, he followed their wishes. After he graduated from dental school, he went into private practice and for almost twenty-five years was quite successful by society's standards. He married his college sweetheart, had three children, built his dream home, and traveled. Still, he never really loved his work; he never felt a great passion for how he spent his days. In one of the counseling sessions he had with me as his holistic lifestyle coach, he told me how much he loved to work in his garden. He even said that if he had to do it all over again, he would go to school and learn to be a landscape architect. So I asked him what was stopping him. He said he could never afford to keep up his current lifestyle if he gave up his practice. I asked him what was more important—happiness or keeping up appearances? I also reminded him that prosperity is an inside job. I gave him a copy of my audio programs *Choose to Live a Balanced Life, How to Achieve Any Goal,* and *Make Your Life a Great Adventure* as well as my book *The Joy Factor.* He began taking night classes in horticulture, gardening, and landscaping and, after three years, got his degree. With a partner, he opened a landscaping business. At the same time, by entering into a partnership with three other dentists, he was able to cut back his dental office time to just two days a week. He discovered that working twice a week as a dentist made him look forward to his work; he knew he was offering a valuable service to his patients. Meanwhile, he put in two to three days a week at his landscaping business, experiencing joy and thoroughly loving being outdoors, creating, and having more time to spend with his family. What's more, he was bringing in more money than he had in his full-time dental practice.

Maybe it's time to take a close look at your line of work. Do you look forward to going to work each day, or do you wish you were doing something different? Sometimes it just takes a change of attitude to make your current job more fulfilling. Listen to your heart. Talk to God and ask for guidance. Pay close attention to the answers you get, and be willing to respond.

Spirit can only do for you what it can do through you. So you must release all obstructions, blockages, and interferences that keep you from God's kingdom. Release everything that has caused you fear, anger, frustration, depression, guilt, shame, and hurt. Through some inner exploration, you'll probably discover that most negative emotions can be traced to your wrong thoughts, wrong words, and wrong actions. In the book *A Spiritual Philosophy for the New World,* author John Price writes: "It is a law of the Universe that whatever you surrender to Spirit is always purified, thus unblocking Spirit's avenues of expression through consciousness." Rather than affirm your way out of a situation, why not simply give it up?

Open your doors and let the light shine through. Become an open receptacle to receive God's gifts of prosperity, abundance, and peace. Give to someone or some organization that inspires and uplifts you. (On my website, under the Contact header, I talk about MVPs and my *Simply*

Radiant programs. That's one option for tithing to a worthy cause.) Love what you do. Listen to your heart. Know that you deserve to be prosperous and that everything you need to live at your highest potential is within you right now. Claim and accept it.

Choose to be prosperous and to attract abundance.

$$\sim$$

Whether people are fully conscious of this or not, they actually derive countenance and sustenance from the "atmosphere" of the things they live in and with.

—FRANK LLOYD WRIGHT

Taking the first footstep with a good thought, the second with a good word, and the third with a good deed, I entered Paradise.

—ZOROASTER

Today's Affirmation & Action Step

I am consciously aware of the spirit of Love within as my source, supply, and support. I deserve to prosper. The more I give of my money or myself, the more I prosper. I am connected to an unlimited source of abundance. My prosperity is coming to me now, and I give thanks.

Tithe your money today to a worthy person or organization. Do it with a loving heart. You might also prefer to put some money in an envelope and leave it at the door of someone you know who's going through a tough time. All you need to say is: "From someone who cares about you and appreciates you." Think prosperous thoughts today.

Day 21

Cultivate a Daily Routine of Living Faithfully

No one can make you feel inferior without your consent.
—ELEANOR ROOSEVELT

We could never learn to be brave and patient if there were only joy in the world.
—HELEN KELLER

Faith, as usually understood, is an elusive quality. The definition in *Webster's* reads, "unquestioning belief that does not require proof or evidence." I see faith not so much as trusting that events will always occur to our liking, but rather trusting that whatever life brings us, our inner resources will rise to the moment and we will be able to handle it. You may have heard the saying "We'll see it when we believe it." Easier said than done, right? It seems to me that, for our faith to truly take hold, we must trust in something greater than ourselves. We must put our trust in Spirit. It is an illusion to believe that any security can be found on Earth; the only security comes from trusting in the Higher Power within you. Through this trust, all things are possible. Trust and faith can work miracles.

In the relatively new field of science of psychoneuroimmunology, researchers are discovering that belief and faith play a major role in healing the body. Psychoneuroimmunological studies show an undeniable link between the workings of the mind, the nervous system, and the body's ability to fight off disease. Studies also reveal that attitudes are based in biochemical realities. Medical research has demonstrated, for example, that panic, depression, hate, fear, and frustration can have negative effects on your health. On the other hand, Norman Cousins presents evidence in his book *Head First: The Biology of Hope* that hope, faith, love, laughter, festivity, the will to live, and a sense of purpose can combat disease.

Faith will lift all sense of discouragement, defeat, and helplessness. Nurturing faith will change your consciousness so that the creative flow of life, love, and unlimited possibilities can fill your being. We cannot expect to see changes in our outer world without first making changes within. We must stop looking outside ourselves for the answers, and instead put all trust in a Higher Power.

We live in a friendly Universe that is always saying yes to us. Our responsibility is to identify and transform the beliefs that have been sabotaging our ability to accept and receive the good that is our birthright. We must learn to trust and love ourselves as much as our Creator does. *When you remove all blockages to the Loving Presence within you and align with the love that you are, abundance, prosperity, peace, and success will be yours.* Believe in yourself. Have faith that nothing is impossible.

There are many people who write off amazing occurrences as coincidences. I don't believe in coincidence. Have you heard the saying "A coincidence is when God decides to do something but prefers to stay anonymous"? I have a story to share with you that I don't think was simply a random happening. In the 1970s, I ran my first marathon in December in Culver City (in the Los Angeles area). I had devoted a year to training. When the race day arrived, I had mixed emotions. On the one hand, I was eager and excited to run, although not quite sure what to expect since I had never done this before. On the other hand, I was feeling sad. The day of the race was the one-year anniversary of my grandmother Fritzie's death. Fritzie, as you know, had been instrumental in teaching me about my own spirituality, self-reliance, simplicity, natural remedies, and about living fully. The morning of the race, I felt a tremendous longing to visit with her. I missed her so much. In the car, I was actually talking out loud with her as a way to soothe my heart. I even told her I was open to her spirit and energy. I asked her to let me know somehow if she could hear me. I asked her to help me through the marathon.

When I arrived at the race site, there were lots of people getting ready. I was wishing I knew someone so I wouldn't have to run alone. The gun went off and so did a few thousand runners. For the first three miles, I was alone and felt great—confident, relaxed, and energetic. Around the fourth mile, a young man who looked to be in his mid-twenties ran up next to me, and we began talking. Before we knew it, we were at mile ten, then fifteen, then twenty. It's amazing the things you'll tell someone you've never met when you're running together. We talked about our lives, families, interests, dreams, and goals. I was extremely grateful to him because our conversation made the miles sail by.

Before we knew it, we were at mile twenty-five. At this point in our conversation, we started talking about where we lived. I told him I lived in Brentwood, and he told me he lived in Studio City. "That's interesting," I said. "My grandmother used to live in Studio City. What street do you live on?" When he told me the street, I gasped, for it was the same street as Fritzie. At this point, we were close to the finish line. I had just enough time to inquire about his exact location. We were crossing the finish line when he told me he had moved into his home eleven months earlier, and that the lady who had lived there before him had passed away. I could hardly breathe, not because I was tired, but because of what he was telling me. He had moved into Fritzie's house!

Coincidence, you say? I don't think so. Out of all the thousands of people in the race, how did I end up running with the man who lived in my grandmother's home? And how do you explain this happening only a few hours after I had asked Fritzie to give me some sign that she was receiving my communication?

Believe. Have faith. Trust your inner guidance. Know you are a cocreator with God and, with that partnership, anything and everything is possible. Relinquish limited thinking. The world is yours for the asking.

Cultivate a daily routine of living faithfully.

~

Enjoying those things for which we were presumably designed in the first place . . . the opportunity to do good work, to fall in love, to enjoy friends, to sit under trees, to read, to hit a ball, to bounce a baby.

—ALISTAIR COOKE

We must be willing to get rid of the life we've planned, so as to have the life that is waiting for us.

—JOSEPH CAMPBELL

Today's Affirmation & Action Step

The spirit of God within is my source, supply, and support. I draw forth the kingdom into my consciousness, and the fullness of my blessings is now being made evident in my world. I stand firm in my faith. Miracles are a natural part of my life. I trust, and I believe.

Today, live with faith that everything is happening and unfolding for your highest good. As each hour arrives, say thank you for everything from the previous hour and for the upcoming hour because you live with a grateful heart and trust in the entire course of things. Living with faith is the gateway to miracles and walking on air. Live faithfully today.

Day 22

Celebrate Your Inherent Intuition

Let us be silent that we may hear the whispers of God.

—RALPH WALDO EMERSON

The Mind's internal heaven shall shed her dews of inspiration on the humblest day.

—WILLIAM WORDSWORTH

Have you ever been thinking of someone you haven't heard from in a long time when suddenly that person called? Did you ever have the feeling that a friend was in trouble, contact him, and find out that he needed your help? Or have you ever met someone and somehow known that this person was going to be your spouse? Some call it a sixth sense, a hunch, a gut feeling, going on instinct, or just knowing deep inside. Psychologists call it intuition—an obscure mental function that provides us with information so that we know without knowing how we know. I refer to it as God's whispering to us and giving us direction.

How tuned in are you to this voice within? I have found from countless experiences that the more we pay attention to our intuition, the more we'll find ourselves in the right place at the right time. Here's a case in point: A few years ago, I was driving around Santa Monica doing some errands. I passed by a quaint little café and, although I wasn't hungry, I felt I should go in and get something to eat. The café wasn't crowded;

only four other tables were occupied. I ordered a salad. Just as it arrived at my table, I noticed the man sitting next to me grabbing his throat. His face was turning red. I knew he was choking. Since I am trained as an emergency medical technician, I quickly went over and asked if he could talk or breathe. He said no and gestured to me that some food was lodged in his throat. I immediately stood him up and performed the Heimlich maneuver. Out popped the food. While all this was happening, the other patrons of the café just watched in disbelief. They applauded when it was over. I think I received more hugs that day than I usually do in a week. Most important, however, I learned how valuable it is to pay attention to and then act on your intuition. I have no doubt that God was making sure I was in the right place at the right time.

The key here is not just getting the message, but listening to it and then acting on it. According to one study I perused recently, divorced couples were asked when they first realized the relationship wasn't going to work out, and an astounding 80 percent replied, "Before the wedding." Although something told them that the marriage was foolhardy, each couple stood together at the altar, either because they wished too strongly that their intuition was wrong or they didn't identify the messages as a kind of knowing they could trust.

I consider myself very intuitive because I have worked for years on developing that faculty. There are a few people in my life who afford me the opportunity to see my intuitive side in action. My dear friend Helen Guppy, who lives in another state, is always picking up on my energy. We might not have talked for three weeks when I'll sit down to write her a letter. Before the letter is complete, she'll call to say hello. Or I'll get an inner signal to call her just when she's thinking of something she needs to ask me. I was the same way with my mother, who was my best friend. We were always picking up on each other's thoughts and feelings even though we were thousands of miles apart, if I was traveling. I'd get a signal that mom was nonplussed about something and I was supposed to call her. When I did, I'd usually find out she was hoping I'd call. It can be quite enjoyable to let your intuition be your guide. People often change their lives not based on what they know, but based on what they feel. When we listen to that inner voice, we are never wrong. The key is really tuning in and paying close attention.

So how can we develop the intuitive side of our being? The best way is just to sit still and listen. Too often, we run away from ourselves, filling up our lives with constant activity. Turn within. Creative geniuses often report that their real-world discoveries are made from connecting to a deep silence within. When someone asked William Blake where he got his ideas, he replied that he stuck his finger through the floor of Heaven and pulled them down. And Michelangelo turned away the congratulations someone proffered him for turning a block of stone into a man, saying the man had been in there all the time and just required a little help in getting out.

Intuition can be nurtured in a variety of ways—through prayer, contemplation, walks in nature, or time spent alone gazing out a window and thinking. Part of receiving these inner messages means learning to give up the analyzing, reasoning, doubting, and limiting part of your mind. And the more you act on your intuitive hunches, the stronger and more readily available they become. As you become more sensitive to your oneness with Infinite Life, you will become more intuitive.

Tuning in to yourself is the basis for becoming all that you were created to be—your best self. As Dag Hammarskjöld, former secretary general of the United Nations, observed, "What you have to attempt [is] to be yourself, to become a mirror in which, according to the degree of purity of heart you have attained, the greatness of life will be reflected."

I would like to end with one of my favorite sayings from Helen Keller. "The most beautiful things in the world cannot be seen or even touched. They must be felt with the heart."

Cultivate your inherent intuition.

~

The one essential thing is that we strive to have light in ourselves.

—ALBERT SCHWEITZER

Even the sun and stars borrow light from the light of consciousness. The Self shining.

—SAINT TERESA OF AVILA

Today's Affirmation & Action Step

*I am a clear and open channel for the power of love to flow through
me. In quietness and confidence, I wait for my guidance. I listen to my
intuition and act on what I hear.*

Pay attention to your inner guidance system—your intuition. When
you get a hunch about something, act on it. Be quiet enough to listen
to and honor your inner whisperings. Think intuitively today.

Day 23

Choose to Lighten Up and Be Childlike

Cannot we let people be themselves, and enjoy life in their own way?
—RALPH WALDO EMERSON

The most wasted day of all is that on which we have not laughed.
—NICOLAS CHAMFORT

When we are anchored in God, no matter what comes our way, we can remain positive and look for the good in everything. Easier said than done, right? Attitude makes all the difference. A positive attitude doesn't just happen by itself; we must cultivate it. William James, the noted philosopher, put it beautifully when he said that the greatest discovery of our generation is that a human being can alter his life by altering his attitude.

Indeed, situations will arise in our lives that may seem difficult, but a positive attitude regards problems as opportunities for growth. I believe that nothing happens that does not afford us the chance to deepen our understanding of and appreciation for life.

A negative attitude functions like an insulator that inhibits the flow of creative energy. Criticism, gossip, anger, fear, envy, suspicion, jealousy, worry, hate, doubt, laziness, anxiety, guilt, and shame are all forms of negative thinking. Watch your thoughts. Make them obey you. Train your mind to think constructively at all times. A joyful, thankful attitude will carry you a long way toward the goal of bringing into your life the health, happiness, and peace that you deserve.

It's been my experience that if you laugh and smile more, your attitude will tilt toward the positive. And if, by chance, you feel you don't have any reason to smile, let me give you four: it firms your facial muscles, it makes you feel better, it makes people wonder what you've been up to, and it creates the quickest bond between two people. And here's a fifth reason from Mother Teresa: "A smile is the beginning of peace."

Humor and laughter have both been found to be important components of healing. William Fry of Stanford University has reported that laughter aids digestion, stimulates the heart, strengthens muscles, activates the brain's creative function, and keeps you alert. So make up your mind to laugh and to be happy. As Abraham Lincoln said, "Most folks are about as happy as they make up their minds to be."

Laughter also helps you keep things in better perspective. When you laugh at yourself, you take yourself far less seriously. "Angels fly because they take themselves lightly," says an old Scottish proverb. Isn't that wonderful?

So with the right attitude, with joy in your heart, with a smile on your face, and a guard at the door of your mind, you can experience life as a great adventure, a celebration of Spirit manifested everywhere. You'll come to realize that life is meant to be lived with a childlike sense of wonder and expectancy. It's not too late to experience life fully. As long as you're breathing, it's never too late.

With your new positive attitude, you will come to understand that it is not the times, the complications of society, or other people that cause problems. It is only your inability to cope. Whatever is going on with you at the moment, choose to make it okay. Give up the fear of making mistakes and the need for approval from others. I see so many people living according to how others expect them to be. Live more from inner guidance. Understand that there is no absolute way to happiness. Rather, acting with happiness is the way.

Being Childlike

So many of us are searching for the fountain of youth—the secret that will enable us to live long and healthy lives. We have tried special diets, supplements, and exercise. Yet, the secret to living a quality life full of vitality and celebration comes from within—from our attitudes, our expressions, and how we view ourselves and the world around us.

Young children are my greatest teachers. They laugh, tell jokes, play, sing, dance, move, and live in their own magical world. They express pure joy. There are no masks when they relate to each other. When children meet for the first time, they often relate as if they were lifetime buddies.

Compare this to your response when meeting someone new. Are you trusting, comfortable, and enthusiastic? Or perhaps suspicious, reserved, and unwilling to be vulnerable? Our individual attitudes and feelings about ourselves are reflected in our actions toward others. Every day we have an opportunity to spread joy in this world by how we relate to other people. It could be something as simple as being a good listener or offering a warm hug. The other person receives your joy and will then pass it along to others. It's so simple and yet so profound. What you give always comes back multiplied.

From my point of view, natural childlike qualities are the true essence of life. They are the magic we should seek to recapture. To be childlike is to be innocent of all the strange, authoritarian ideas of what adulthood ought to be. Children are trusting and straightforward, honest and natural, free from the need to impress others. Being childlike means being more concerned with the experiences of life than with how others view you. You do not have to give up being an adult in order to become more childlike. You do not have to become infantile or irresponsible or unaccountable. The fully integrated person is capable of harmoniously blending the adult and the child.

Think about the adults you most like to be with. I'll bet they are genuinely happy, joyful people. From joyfulness flows laughter, a sense of humanness, and silliness. You don't always have to be orderly, rigid, serious, and adultlike. Learn to have fun and to be a little silly and crazy. In other words, lighten up. When you do this, the whole world will seem brighter and more beautiful.

Within each of us is a child waiting to come forth and express himself or herself more fully. What usually keeps us from getting in touch with the child within is our unwillingness to recognize and accept this child. We often feel that we have to act our age. But our happiness relies on our ability to recover the vibrancy and spontaneity that may be missing in our life. Remember to laugh, simplify your life, slow down, take time to smell the flowers, talk to the animals, watch the clouds, enjoy a sunrise and sunset.

In my life, I have noticed that when my judgmental self rears its ugly head, I tend to be more controlling instead of letting go and flowing with life. When I release my desire to be in control and to live more from inner guidance, I notice that struggle dissipates and I feel more peaceful.

The more I pay attention to how children experience and embrace life, and the more I release my fears about feeling uncertain, the better life becomes because the more gentle, tenderhearted parts of me come forward. As that happens, the oppositions within my life soften. My work becomes play; my challenges become wonderful opportunities to learn and to grow. My life takes on clarity and purpose as I move closer to becoming a master at the art of living.

Each day, make a point of doing something out of the ordinary that brings joy to others and to you. The results may surprise you. For example, I love teddy bears. Often when I take long trips in my car, my bears accompany me. I also take one when I fly, tucked snugly in my carry-on bag, or sitting next to me if the seat is empty. My bears help me keep my inner child alive and happy.

Children accept your good points and your not-so-good points. They don't care about differences, about different races, religions, or backgrounds. In a world in which so much conflict exists, the best bridge to understanding, peace, and joy is built through love and forgiveness. When we reach out to another and offer unconditional love and forgiveness, as children do, joy and peace are the result.

Choose to lighten up and be childlike.

∾

Living well means putting a big emphasis on having some fun.

—ALEXANDRA STODDARD

Bless the good-natured, for they bless everybody else.

—Thomas Carlyle

Today's Affirmation & Action Step

I choose to let my inner child come out and orchestrate my day. I greet each day with joy in my heart and laughter in my eyes. I love my life and know that everything is in divine order.

At some point today, do something that brings out your inner child. For example, if you drive by a children's playground, stop and swing on the swing set. Or fly a kite, throw a Frisbee, or skip during your daily walk. As you're doing this out-of-the-ordinary activity, feel your inner child coming out to play. Be more childlike today.

Day 24

Cultivate the Delight of Self-Reliance and Detachment

Self-reliance, the height and perfection of man, is reliance on God.
—RALPH WALDO EMERSON

How to gain, how to keep, how to recover happiness is . . . for most people at all times the secret motive of all they do.
—WILLIAM JAMES

I learned more about self-reliance from my grandmother Fritzie and my mom June than from anyone else in my life. I wish you could have known them. They were both spirited, happy, shining souls who celebrated life every day. They loved to travel and did so often. Fritzie traveled all over the world, usually alone, too. She took very little with her, just a few basics. She wanted to live simply. Both my mom and grandmother were never afraid to visit new places, and they always made friends wherever they went.

Living alone was important to Fritzie. When I asked her if she ever got lonely, she responded by saying. "Heavens, no! How could I possibly get lonely when God is always with me?" That response led to a long discussion about independence, self-reliance, and faith in God that profoundly affected my life.

American psychologist Abraham Maslow characterized his healthiest subjects as independent, detached, and self-governing, with a tendency to look within for their guiding values and for the rules by which they live. He also noted their strong preference, even need, for privacy and their detachment from people in general. My grandmother certainly fits Maslow's description of a healthy person. Maslow discovered that his healthiest subjects were only superficially accepting of social customs, while in private they were quite casual about and even humorously tolerant of them. These people defied convention when they thought it necessary and judged things by their own criteria. They lived by their own values, not the dictates of society. Maslow called such people "autonomous."

For more than ten years now, I have been living my life autonomously. I spend a great deal of my time alone, and I go to great lengths to protect my privacy and solitude. Sure, I love being with people and, in my work, I come in contact with several thousand people per year. Yet, when I'm not with others, I love to spend quality time by myself. In fact, on a regular basis, I detach myself from the world and spend time alone. It's true freedom to feel the peace of your own company. I've had friends who didn't understand my desire for solitude. As a result, the friendships have dissolved, and new and more fulfilling ones have entered my life.

To be self-reliant means you become centered in that bedrock of wholeness inside you. Detach from those things that limit and weaken you and become one with those that empower you. Self-reliance, as Emerson suggests, means relying not on our Lower Selves but instead on our Higher Selves.

Too often in relationships, we rely on the other person to make us feel good or to guarantee our self-confidence. As my mom and grandmother used to teach me, the goal of life is to move from the support of the environment to self-support—and striving to go deeper within ourselves.

Have you considered that most of us grow up believing that what others say is more important than what we think or how we feel? We've been conditioned to look outside ourselves to establish our self-esteem. From my counseling work, I have learned that people emphasize what they *do* (instead of who they are) in order to determine how "good" they are. We become too attached to valuing others' opinions. I've seen this principle in my own career. I used to be concerned that my articles or seminars were well received. But when I chose to give up that worry and to speak and write more from my heart, I found that not only did I do much better, I also began receiving a deluge of offers to write and speak. I allowed myself to work knowing that the outcome isn't the most essential thing.

A Western journalist once asked Gandhi, "Can you give me the secret of your life in three words?" Gandhi replied, "Renounce and enjoy!" With a more detached attitude, we can flow through life without judgment about how things are supposed to be. We see that it's the heart we carry within us and the peace we feel that foster fulfillment. Don't be attached to a specific outcome. With this open attitude, you can become centered and allow the divine flow to see you through.

Detachment releases joy and is the secret to peace of mind. When I began this 30-day rejuvenation and writing process, part of my surrender was letting go of all the things and people in my life, knowing they were safe in God's hands. I wanted to detach from the outside world so I could become truly anchored in the divine. Through this process, I've realized that detachment has more to do with what we think and feel and less to do with our actions. I needed to become detached from my judgment about the way things should be and more in alignment with how God wants things to be. This realization made me feel free and light. Practicing detachment takes away stress and thus fosters greater health. You become less preoccupied with the things of the earth and more focused on God's plan for you. This is true self-reliance—knowing you already have everything you need to live fully.

Choose the delight of self-reliance and detachment.

∼

Make your life something beautiful for God.

—MOTHER TERESA

*What is your purpose, what is your calling? What I know for
sure is, if you ask the question the answer will come. You have
to be willing to listen for the answer. You have to get still enough
to learn it and hear it and pay attention, to be fully conscious
enough to see not just with your eyes but through them to the
truth of who you are and what you can be.*

—OPRAH WINFREY

Today's Affirmation & Action Step

*I put my reliance in the wisdom and the love within me, and I know that
my life is now in divine order. My happiness comes from my heart, and I
detach from living my life according to the dictates of others. In all things
and in all ways, I follow my heart.*

Live without any judgments throughout this day. When you feel
a judgment rearing its ugly head, cancel it immediately. Say aloud
or silently, "Cancel," and then replace the thought with a positive,
enriching thought. And then smile because you're aware of changing
your negative patterns. Detach yourself from negativity. Think happy,
uplifting thoughts today.

Day 25

Celebrate Your Relationships

In about the same degree as you are helpful you will be happy.

—THEODOR REIK

The highest service we can perform for others is to help them help themselves.

—HORACE MANN

One of the great joys in life comes from the relationships we form with others. At the same time, relationships can also present some of our greatest challenges.

To experience harmony in our relationships, we must learn to see and love the divine in others and understand that lasting relationships result from *being* the right person, not *finding* the right person. A basic spiritual principle is that there is only oneness: we are all one with everyone and everything we encounter. Instead of trying to change or fix someone whom we see as the source of problems or difficulties, we can remind ourselves who that person really is. Instead of focusing on outer appearance and behavior—quirks, idiosyncrasies, clothes, hairstyles—we can look at one another with the thought, "That is a soul, a child of God. That human being is an expression of the Infinite." By doing so, we acquire greater understanding and new perspective: that person has feelings, just as I do. She has thoughts and opinions, aspirations and dreams that are just as important to her as mine are to me. The life force of God in that person is manifesting in her personality, in the services she performs, in the way she treats others, and in her whole way of being. Because I know who I am, a divine child of God, I can focus on the divinity in others.

As you absorb this higher image of who you are, many wonderful benefits follow. You no longer relate to yourself as a creature whose satisfaction comes solely from physical pleasures. You stop relating to others in terms of their physical appearance. Because you know that your worth derives from the eternal self within you, and because you know that this same self lives in the hearts of all, you relate to everyone with respect, kindness, and love, no matter the circumstance.

This change of attitude is one of the most joyful benefits of spiritual experience, yet it brings enormous responsibilities. In order to see ourselves in all others, we must become detached from our own ego. Otherwise, we will get emotionally entangled in other people's problems and lose sight of our oneness with Spirit. You must practice detachment if you want to create loving, harmonious relationships. Being spiritually detached means being a very loving person. It also means being able to stand back and let go of your own needs and preferences. Without this detachment, you cannot help but manipulate other people, which will only create conflict in your relationships.

Peace comes from practicing detachment continuously—at home, at work, with friends and relatives, and especially with difficult people. A spiritually detached person will not let a relationship degenerate to provocation and response. The test is simple: Even if you are upset or angry with me, can I remain calm, loving, and kind with you and help you overcome your anger? If you persist in being upset with me, can I still act lovingly toward you?

A dislike for people is really a reflection on us rather than on those we do not like. We tend to see others not as they really are, but as we are. Our relationships are always mirrors, reflecting some aspect of ourselves. Pay close attention when a particular pattern is mirrored back from three or more different people. To an angry person, everyone seems angry and full of hostility. To a suspicious person, everybody seems suspect. To a loving, tenderhearted person, everybody is worthy of love; every occasion is an opportunity to see the best in the other person.

I'm not saying that if you are loving and detached, you'll never experience difficulty in relationships. People will still get angry or fail to treat you nicely. And with people who treat us unkindly and disrespectfully, we must look harder to see the divine in them. There may be relationships that are unhealthy and abusive. In those instances, you usually need to remove yourself from the environment while both of you get help. Still, you can love that other person (although you don't have to love his behavior) and put him in the hands of Love. As I'll write about next, forgiveness is also part of this process.

With practice and commitment to your own divinity, you will see that people will begin to come around. Being around someone who is loving, gentle, tender, and peaceful softens others' hearts. And when we bring to a relationship our awareness of our own divinity and keep our hearts open, it is amazing how people's attitudes toward us change.

If we want to get along with others, we should not treat people as objects, but as human beings who are children of the Light, and deserving of our love and peace. I once heard Buckminster Fuller say, "We are not nouns, we are verbs." People who have rigid images of others think of themselves and their fellow human beings as nouns, or as things. Those who keep the awareness of their oneness close at hand and strive to understand and appreciate others more behave more like verbs— enthusiastic, open, active, creative, able to change themselves and to make changes in the world. They keep one goal in mind: to identify and remove all the blockages to the awareness of Spirit's presence in everything and everyone, including themselves.

Everyone wants to feel loved, appreciated, nurtured, and supported. This is particularly true for children and teenagers. Our role as parents is to support, guide, and nurture them and to provide an environment in which our children experience high self-esteem and are free to discover their God-given talents. Too often we are tempted to manipulate or coerce them into doing what we think they ought to be doing. We need to trust that the Infinite is revealing its highest vision to our children. We must help our children believe in themselves and live their vision. Remember, our children are not here to fulfill our unrealized dreams, nor do they exist to help us resolve all of our unfinished business. They are God's children, and Spirit already has a wonderful journey prepared for them. Our role is to love them unconditionally, to support and guide them, and to help them realize how capable they are. To do this, we must feel lovable, capable, and worthy ourselves.

Children reflect the consciousness of their parents. When your children are causing problems, look at what needs adjusting in your own life. Case in point: Last month, I went to the movies with a friend and his teenage daughter. When my friend purchased the tickets, although he should have paid the adult price for all of us (his daughter was thirteen), he said, "Two adults and one child." Just a few days prior, he had been talking with his daughter about the importance of always telling the truth. Which message do you think spoke more loudly to her?

In my counseling practice, people often come to me wanting advice on how to discipline their problem children. Before I address that question, I first look at the parents, how they feel about themselves, and what values and attitudes they are conveying to their children. Until we deal with our own consciousness and take care of unfinished business, all of our attempts to "fix" a problem child are only going to compound the situation. In every situation, whether the relationship is with a child or an adult, I ask myself, "What is this situation telling me about myself? What is this challenge revealing to me? How can I be more loving to the other person?" I know that if I can raise my consciousness to the level of the heart-light within me, especially in the most difficult and trying times, then I will be able to see more clearly, to respond instead of react, and to resolve differences instead of increasing conflict.

It's been my experience in my counseling work with all kinds of relationships that problems usually escalate when the spiritual element is not present in a relationship. When we feel separate from our spiritual selves, we become more fearful and try to control everything. We listen to the voice of the ego, and what we hear is how to live more fearfully. Letting go of negative thoughts and removing fear improves dealings with individuals in every area of life. If a relationship is truly a giving one, a couple will decide together to be gentle and kind to everyone they see.

Demonstrating peace, kindness, love, and gentleness in daily life means having a loving connection not just to another person, but to ourselves as well, which means surrendering ourselves to God and seeing God in all our relationships. One of the greatest gifts you can give is to help others experience themselves as beautiful, lovable, capable, and deserving.

Something happened yesterday that reminded me I have a ways to go in my effort to establish loving relationships with everyone. I was talking to a close friend on the telephone. He is usually very tenderhearted and kind with me, and that shows in his voice and his way of being. But yesterday morning was different; he sounded distant, cold, and harsh. He was frustrated with work, he was fighting off a cold, and he wanted to clarify a plan we were making for a special celebration. Instead of responding to him with love and tenderness, I reacted by saying, "Well, there's no need to be so mean and harsh; maybe we should talk about this another time when you're in a better mood." As you can imagine, that only upset him more and distanced him further. He became more hostile, and I felt ready to give up. Trying to see the divinity in this man was the furthest thing from my mind. We got off the telephone saying we were both okay, even though neither of us meant it.

I thought all day about that phone conversation. I realized that I was too attached to the way I expected my friend to be. I was unwilling to acknowledge that anyone can have a bad day. I didn't have to take his attitude as a personal attack. I could, instead, choose to offer my understanding and patience. After an entire day went by, I finally got brave enough to call and apologize for my behavior. I told him I would work on being more understanding and loving and wouldn't take his distancing mood changes personally. At the same time, he acknowledged that he didn't need to take out his frustrations with work on me and, because he cared for me so much and knows how much I value others being tenderhearted and loving, he would work on his behavior and attitude. All in all, through communication and a willingness to move forward, we were able to resolve the conflict and come closer together in spirit.

I like to think that God's harp strings connect all hearts. When we choose to distance ourselves from others, some of those harp strings break, and the music we hear is no longer harmonious. When we choose to see the divine in everyone and to respond lovingly no matter how someone else treats us, then we create beautiful music.

I'd like to end with one of my favorite quotes from Gerald Jampolsky's book *Out of the Darkness, Into the Light:* "Our purpose in relationships is just to see that spirit of love in each other, the light of love in everyone. That is the only reality."

Celebrate your relationships.

~

Nothing here below is profane for those who know how to see.

—Pierre Teilhard de Chardin

Love . . . delights in what it looks at; and at its purest, it recognizes no higher purpose than delight.

—Deepak Chopra

Today's Affirmation & Action Steps

I know that the essence of my being is love, and I choose to extend this love to everyone in my life. Regardless of outer circumstances, I remain peaceful and tenderhearted. I love myself and others unconditionally and know that we are all children of God. In our oneness, I see divinity in everything and everyone.

Write or call three people today and let them know how important and special they are to you. It will color their day positively and will make you feel good, too. Think happy relationships today.

Day 26

Choose to Forgive

One kind word can warm three winter months.

—Japanese Saying

*When you hold resentment against anyone, you are bound to
that person by a cosmic link, a real tough mental chain. You are
tied by a cosmic tie to the thing that you hate. The one person,
perhaps in the whole world, whom you most dislike, is the
very one to whom you are attracting yourself, by a hook that is
stronger than steel.*

—Emmet Fox

Forgiveness changes lives. Choosing to forgive unlocks the gate to healing and health, prosperity and abundance, joy and happiness, and inner peace. As we learned in previous chapters, patience can be essential to this process, but with faith, you can always come to a place of new understanding and forgiveness. Jesus said, "Father, forgive them for they know not what they do" (Luke 23:34). He also told His disciples, "Whenever you stand praying, forgive, if you have anything against anyone, so that your Father who also is in heaven may forgive you your trespasses" (Mark 11:24–25). The Master always reinforced the need for forgiveness.

Forgiveness is the central teaching of many of the world's religions. Forgiveness can heal our minds, dispel our pain, and ultimately awaken us from the confines of time and space. It's the vehicle that helps us to release fear and the past. To forgive is to let go. Forgiveness lightens our hearts and reunites them with the divine. Through forgiveness, miracles occur.

As so aptly stated by Emmet Fox at the beginning of this chapter, you become linked to another person when you don't offer forgiveness. You also give away your power by creating a charged, emotionally active connection. But when you forgive, you take back your power and can no longer be controlled by the other person. Some say that forgiveness is a sign of weakness. I disagree. It takes strength and a generous spirit to understand that people do not always hurt us because they choose to, but more because they couldn't help it. People do harm to others when they are in pain or are out of alignment with their source. If you give back to another person the same pain that person has given you, you are making it impossible for a miracle to occur.

You can transform any negative emotion into love. Though you can't control another person's feelings, you can choose what you want to experience, and how you want to be. Let kindness and tenderheartedness be your goal. Jesus tells us to love our enemies. I understand how difficult this can be, especially when you believe someone has wronged you. Maybe you ask yourself, "How can I forgive what this person has done to me?" The secret is to get out of the way and let the Loving Presence forgive through you. "To err is human, to forgive divine," wrote Alexander Pope. When you choose to live your life more internally, your heart softens and your life changes. Resentments, anger, guilt, and hurt are released. But you can't release these negative emotions yourself. In my prayer time every day, I ask God to show me how to forgive the past, forgive others, and forgive myself.

Forgiveness has to start with the self. Be gentle. When we forgive ourselves, that doesn't mean we condone everything we have done. It means we claim it and own it. We accept that we made some mistakes and now it's time to let go and to move on. Let go. Release all the pain and replace it with God's love. When you forgive yourself, you move more fully back into your heart.

Forgiveness is also an essential ingredient in any healthy, successful relationship. Communication is the key. Be aware of your feelings and allow them to come to the surface for you to own. Share these feelings with your partner. Never go to sleep feeling angry, resentful, or upset. Offer forgiveness, let go, and let Love purify your emotions.

What if you can't contact another person or that other person has passed away? It doesn't matter. Forgiveness means a change of heart. It was about twenty years after my dad had passed away that I forgave him for what I believed he had done to me as a child. I also forgave myself for having unloving thoughts about my dad. God showed me the way to do these things. I wrote my dad a letter, I visited his gravesite, and I brought him to my mind's eye and talked with him. As a result of practicing forgiveness with my dad, miracles occurred—in my relationships, in my career, and in my health. And from this forgiveness, I experienced a profound peace. There's no doubt in my mind that forgiveness is the greatest act of healing; it transforms lives, and it creates miracles.

Choose to forgive.

~

Kind words produce their own image in men's souls; and a beautiful image it is.

—Blaise Pascal

No matter what you are doing, keep the undercurrent of happiness. Learn to be secretly happy within your heart in spite of all circumstances.

—Paramahansa Yogananda

Today's Affirmation & Action Step

Forgiveness is a gift I offer others and myself. It acts as my heart's paintbrush and can color anything bright and luminescent. I let the purifying wash of forgiveness cleanse all of my past mistakes and wrong thinking. I now have an inward sense of peace and tranquility.

Offer forgiveness to someone in your life today. You might choose to do it in a note or telephone call or in person. If this person is no longer living, you can still extend forgiveness in the form of a letter. It will release you from the darkness and lift you up into the light of love and peace. Think forgiveness today.

Day 27

Cultivate Courage in Everything

Life is either a daring adventure—or nothing.

—HELEN KELLER

Live your life while you have it. Life is a splendid gift.

—FLORENCE NIGHTINGALE

It takes daring just to live, but it takes courage to live your vision. Is it possible to be in touch with your true courageousness without being in touch with your divinity? I don't think so. We can soar to the top of the mountain and beyond when we know that the courage we want is part of us; this comes from our trust in Love. Trust in the Loving Presence will destroy the fear that stifles our efforts.

Fear means looking through our human eyes and mind rather than through the eyes and the heart of God. When we face our fears, and act from the awareness that we are one with Spirit, we learn and nurture courage. Goethe said, "Whatever you can do, or dream you can, begin it. Boldness has genius, power, and magic in it." When we face our fears head on, they begin to evaporate. When we embrace what scares us, we find that we are endowed with a level of courage that we never knew existed. Every day we have so many opportunities to act courageously. Committing to a 30-day program takes courage. Putting fresh ideas on paper each day takes courage. Getting up each morning to face the day as a willing participant takes courage. Become enthusiastic about your life. Muster the courage to live your life with gusto. It was Thomas

Edison who said: "When a man dies, if he can pass enthusiasm along to his children, he has left them an estate of incalculable value." Let courage be the shield that protects you. In the end, most people don't regret the things they do. They regret what they failed to do.

Why do you defend limitations? Why let fear paralyze you? Choose differently. Let Spirit be your guide, with courage at the reins. My mom taught me to be courageous. She would never allow me to defend my limitations.

What is courage to you? To me, courage means moving through uncertainty. Courage means changing when that's the hardest thing in the world to do. Courage means being responsible for what you've created in life and relinquishing blame. It's making difficult choices when, in this fast-paced, overstimulated world, we're overwhelmed with information. Courage is choosing to live simply when everything seems to teach the opposite. Some people think that if you have courage, you don't have fear. Not at all! Courage is being fearful but doing it anyway, and courage is admitting you don't know all the answers. Courage is trusting again in a relationship, even when you've been hurt or disappointed. Courage is living up to the promises we've made to ourselves and to others. Courage is when we do what we have to do even though we might not want to.

True courage enables us to live in the present and make choices rather than being a victim and settling for what life gives us. Sometimes we just need to make the choice to move in the direction of our dreams. Movement is powerful. The American dancer and choreographer Martha Graham, a premier figure in modern dance who lived to ninety-seven, always advocated movement: "There is a vitality, a life force, an energy, a quickening that is translated through you into action, and because there is only one of you in all time, this expression is unique. And if you block it, it will never exist through any other medium and will be lost." I love that thought.

Too much analyzing and rationalizing can lead to lack of courage. Let your inner child spark your motivation to take some action. I used to hear Buckminster Fuller say in his talks, "Dare to be naïve." Isn't that fantastic! You get an idea, it excites you, it makes you feel wonderful, it benefits you and others, it causes no harm to anyone, and it would be a joy to create in your life. Go for it! Do what it takes.

Believe that you've been given this wish to fulfill and let no one and nothing cause you to doubt your power and ability to make this wish come true. Be just naïve enough to believe that this wish is yours to bring to fruition. Trust in the wish, take the steps necessary to bring it to fruition, and know that you deserve to create your best life. It starts right here, in the present moment.

Several years ago, I went alone to the Sierra Nevada Mountains for a few days of quiet and prayer, and just to be out in nature. On this particular summer trip, I had a cabin next to a beautiful placid lake. My last day there, I decided to take an all-day hike in the mountains. I left at around dawn and hiked uphill for most of the morning. It was unusually quiet that day; I passed only five people on the trails. Around two in the afternoon, I decided to sit down, relax, and meditate by a tree. Sitting cross-legged, with my eyes still open, I could see paradise—several lakes and most of the Sierras. With each breath, I felt more peaceful, relaxed, and connected with the spirit of life. I closed my eyes and began to concentrate on my breath, slowly inhaling and slowly exhaling. It felt wonderful. In a few more moments, I was totally absorbed in my inner world, not at all distracted by my surroundings, except for one minor thing. I thought I could hear some leaves moving. Often, when I'm meditating outdoors, I'm extra sensitive to nature's sounds. I figured I was in tune with the leaves and their musical dance. After a few more minutes, however, the sound of the leaves rustling got louder. Slightly curious, I opened one eye. What I saw made my heart jump so that I thought it was on the outside of my body. No more than about twenty feet in front of me was a bear.

My first reaction was unbridled fear. The bear just stood there and stared at me. My second reaction was to ask God what to do. The answer was instantaneous and, as I look back on the situation, somewhat off the wall. Or should I say the tree? I was told to breathe slowly and deeply— as best I could. I was also told to smile at the bear and to say some kind words from my heart. I gave it my best shot. I told the bear—in a voice three octaves higher than I use for speaking—that he was beautiful, his fur was shiny, and that I didn't intend on being his lunch. By talking to him, I actually began to feel relaxed. As I acted with courage, the fear slowly began to disappear. For about five minutes, I spoke to the bear.

Then something really amazing occurred. I sensed that the bear was talking with me and responding to my comments. He even seemed to smile. Yes, part of me was still scared, but not paralyzed or mentally frozen. I paid attention, felt all my emotions fully, and actually enjoyed the experience. Then the bear started to move in my direction, but I wasn't quite ready to hold out my hand to pet him. Before he got to me, he turned around and shuffled away. As I watched him meander off into the forest, I reflected on my extraordinary experience, one in which I learned that courage is inside of us all just waiting to rear its beautiful head.

We strengthen and develop our courage by using it. Don't let your courage go to waste. Trust in who you are and be all you were created to be by living a courageous life.

Cultivate courage in everything.

～

I always try to check my motivation and be mindful and present in the moment.

—THE DALAI LAMA

Today's Affirmation & Action Step

Courage is my middle name and is part of my very nature. I am courageous in all my activities today and trust that the Spirit within me will show me what to do and what to say. I have the courage to face anything and everything, including myself. I trust the whisperings of my heart to lead me to my very best life.

Is there something you've wanted to do but haven't had the courage to take the first step? Do it today. Whatever it is—calling someone, writing page one of your novel, joining a gym or crafts group, seeking therapy or counseling, or simply going to a movie alone for the first time in your life. Do it. Don't put it off another day. The step of courage you undertake today will springboard you into a more extraordinary life. Think courageous thoughts today.

Day 28

Celebrate Salubrious Silence
and Solitude

Love consists in this, that two solitudes protect and touch and greet each other.
—RAINER MARIA RILKE

Well-timed silence hath more eloquence than speech.
—MARTIN FARQUHAR TUPPER

Noise seems to be part of our everyday lives—from the alarm clock in the morning to the traffic outside to the never-ending sounds of voices, radio, and television. Our bodies and minds appear to have acclimated to these outside intrusions. But have they really?

Over two decades ago, the Committee on Environmental Quality of the Federal Council for Science and Technology found that "a growing number of researchers fear the dangerous and hazardous effects of intense noise on human health are seriously underestimated." Similarly, former vice president Nelson Rockefeller, when writing about the environmental crisis of his time, noted that when people are fully aware of the damage noise can inflict, "peace and quiet will surely rank along with clean skies and pure waters as top priorities for our generation."

More recent studies suggest that our bodies pay a price for adapting to noise: higher blood pressure, heart rate, and adrenaline secretion; heightened aggression; impaired resistance to disease; and a sense of helplessness.

I haven't been able to find many studies on the effects of quiet on repairing the stress of noise, but I know intuitively that most of us love quiet and need it desperately. We've become so accustomed to having noise in our lives that silence can sometimes feel awkward and unsettling. On vacation, for instance, when quiet prevails, we may have trouble sleeping. But choosing times of silence can enrich the quality of our lives tremendously. If you find yourself overworked, stressed out, irritated, or tense, rather than heading for a coffee or snack break, maybe all you need is a silence break.

Everyone at some time has experienced the feeling of being overwhelmed by life. Everyone, too, has felt the need to escape, to find a secluded place to experience the peace of Spirit, to be alone with quiet thoughts. Creating times of silence in our lives takes commitment and discipline. Most of the time, periods of silence must be scheduled into your day's activities or you'll never have this kind of time.

Carve out times of silence while at home. Turn off the radio, television, and telephones. If you live with a family, maybe the best quiet time for you is early in the morning before others rise. In that silence, you can become more aware, more sensitive to your surroundings, and feel more in touch with the wholeness of life.

Recognize the importance of solitude. Silence and solitude go hand in hand. In silence and solitude, you reconnect with your inner self. Solitude helps to clear your channels, fosters peacefulness, and brings spiritual lucidity. When you retreat from the outside world to go within, you can be at the very center of your being and reacquaint yourself with your spiritual nature—the essence of your being and of all life.

Outside noise tends to drown out the inner life—the music of the soul. Only in silence and solitude can we go within and nurture our spiritual lives. This is the harbor of the heart. When you rediscover that harbor, your life will never be the same. In the Bible we read, "There is silence in heaven" (Rev. 8:1). "For God alone my soul waits in silence" (Ps. 62:1).

Mystics, saints, and spiritual leaders have all advocated periods of silence and solitude for spiritual growth. Saint John of the Cross writes that only in silence can the soul hear the Divine. Jesus often prayed by Himself and spent long hours in silent communion with God. Gandhi devoted every Monday to silence. When I read about Gandhi's practice of silence and solitude several years ago, I was so inspired that I decided to adopt a similar discipline in my life. So now one day a week, for two consecutive days once a month, and for several days in a row at each change of season, I spend time in solitude, silence, prayer, and quiet. Even now, during this 30-day rejuvenation program, I have chosen to spend most of my time alone in silence.

How do you feel about being alone? Aloneness is quite different from loneliness. This idea is expressed beautifully by Paul Tillich in *Courage to Be.*

> Our language has wisely sensed the two sides of being alone. It has created the word "loneliness" to express the pain of being alone. And it has created the word "solitude" to express the glory of being alone.

Loneliness is something you do to yourself. Have you ever experienced feeling lonely even when you're with other people? We must reclaim ourselves through reconnection with our wholeness and the peace of solitude. Choose to make solitude your friend.

Even if you're married, you still need times of privacy and solitude. In my counseling, I always encourage couples to spend occasional time alone, not only daily, but also at regular intervals during the week, month, and year. In this way, you regain your identity as individuals. You bring so much more to the marriage when you feel whole, complete, and strong. Solitude fosters these qualities.

With a little creativity, a marriage can accommodate solitude and privacy. I have witnessed all types of arrangements, including separate vacations, private rooms in the house, living separately during the week and coming together on weekends, and having special times during the day in which each person is left alone.

I know several people who do everything possible to preclude being alone. Often, this is because they are afraid of loneliness or are simply uncomfortable with themselves. They haven't yet discovered the peace of their own company. It's not scary to be by yourself; it's absolutely wonderful. Loneliness is not a state of being; it's simply a state of mind. You can choose to change your state of mind.

I realize that I live my life differently from most. I go to great lengths to secure my time of solitude and privacy. It's a great comfort to me to be by myself; it's like returning home to an old friend or a lover after being away too long. Solitude is not a luxury. It is a right and a necessity.

It is my contention that all the good things we endeavor to provide for ourselves, including sound nutrition, daily exercise, and material wealth, will be of reduced value unless we learn to live in harmony with ourselves, which means finding peace in our own company. This peace is a natural result of spending time alone in silence. Of course, in spending time alone we realize that we are never really alone and that we can live more fully by focusing on inner guidance rather than on externalities.

Celebrate salubrious silence and solitude.

$\sim$

It is better to keep your mouth closed and let people think you are a fool than to open it and remove all doubt.

—MARK TWAIN

Walk in silence; go quietly; develop spiritually. We should not allow noise and sensory activities to ruin the antennae of our attention, because we are listening for the footsteps of God to come into our temples.

—PARAMAHANSA YOGANANDA

Today's Affirmation & Action Step

In the silence of my heart, I am at peace. In solitude, I celebrate myself and my life and all its rich blessings. Today I seek out time to be alone, to enjoy the serenity of my own company.

Carve out ten to thirty minutes to be alone and completely silent today. Turn off the TV, radio, and even the ringer on the telephone. If you live with others, or you are at work, let others know that you don't want to be disturbed. This silence and aloneness will enrich your day and week. Think silence today.

Day 29

Choose to Meditate and
to Live Peacefully

We must learn to live together as brothers or perish as fools.
—MARTIN LUTHER KING JR.

*Reading makes a full man, meditation a profound man,
discourse a clear man.*
—BENJAMIN FRANKLIN

Meditation provides numerous benefits for your body; it releases tension, reduces stress and high blood pressure, boosts immune function, improves concentration, increases awareness, and brings about a more positive attitude. But there is so much more to meditation than this. Meditation restores calmness to the mind, so that we can perceive God's reflection in our souls.

The more regularly you meditate, the easier it becomes. Eventually, after years of practicing meditation, you will become one with the rhythm of universal life; then every moment of your life becomes a meditation, a communion with God. This takes self-discipline and commitment.

If none of this jazzes you, maybe this will: scientific studies show that people who meditate regularly have the physiology of someone who's twelve to fifteen years younger. They have fewer wrinkles and a more youthful appearance as a result of feeling less stress and being more at peace from meditating. Now I bet I've got your attention, right?

In prayer, I talk to God. In meditation, I listen to God. It is not a passive exercise, since I am in meditation for inspiration and spiritual revelation. During meditation, I rise in consciousness into an atmosphere of receptivity, into a consciousness in which I feel the Light and all life becomes one. To become centered in the divine consciousness, to me, is the first essential of a fulfilling and peaceful life. As I rest in the divine, in quiet meditation, I feel God's energy flowing through my mind, brain, and nervous system. I am radiant with light. My mind is purified, my body is glorified, and my life is filled with peace and joy.

Meditation brings deep peace, joy, humility, patience, gratefulness, and caring the way nothing else does. Through meditation, I celebrate that special oneness with my source; it's my strength and guiding light. I am very disciplined about this part of my life. I arise early (before sunrise) each morning to meditate. Then before I sleep at night, I meditate again, time permitting.

I encourage everyone to meditate twice a day, beginning with twenty minutes each session. If more people meditate, the effect on the planet will be profound—we will create a more peaceful world. World peace is a function of our collective inner peace. For the whole world to be elevated to a higher level of awareness, all of us must participate.

Meditation is a natural process of turning within. There is nothing to be afraid of, but, of course, it takes practice—disciplined practice. Through regular meditation, we begin to experience our world through new senses; we start to see beyond our old reality, as defined by appearances, and we enter a state of clarity where we share a common bond. We find that inner peace and unconditional love are, in fact, real and in our hearts.

If you are a beginner, I suggest you study more about meditation to get a better understanding of its practice, purpose, and benefits. On my website, I have an audiobook you'll enjoy titled *Wired to Meditate*. It covers everything you need to know to get started on a meditation program or to enrich your existing program. In studying meditation, you will gain some insight, but this should never take the place of meditation itself.

One of the greatest benefits of meditation for me is that I have become very peaceful and, most of the time, can live in a center of peace and serenity regardless of what is going on outside me. In that calmness, I feel my connection with God and know that, with this type of partnership, anything is possible. My life has become a great unfolding adventure and has taken on a richness and profundity that nothing in my outside world could ever provide. I salute your great adventure as well.

Choose to meditate and to live peacefully.

~

This is the true joy in life, the being used for a purpose recognized by yourself as a mighty one.

—GEORGE BERNARD SHAW

Whenever anyone has offended me, I try to raise my soul so high that the offense cannot reach it.

—RENÉ DESCARTES

Today's Affirmation & Action Step

The most important thing in my life is to remember God. In quiet meditation, the Indwelling Presence shows me the way to live in love and peace. My life has become a great adventure, and I'm living fully—healthfully, joyfully, and peacefully.

At some point today, take ten to forty-five minutes to meditate. Focus on your breath, and breathe deeply and slowly. When you find your mind wandering, as it will, gently bring it back to the focus of your breath or an affirmation you silently recite. Some affirmations I use include "I am peaceful" or "I am infused with Love." These few minutes in meditation will enrich and uplift your entire day. Think meditation today.

Day 30

Cultivate Your Very Best Life

Though we travel the world over to find the beautiful, we must carry it with us or we find it not.

—RALPH WALDO EMERSON

The more you lose yourself in something bigger than yourself, the more energy you will have.

—NORMAN VINCENT PEALE

Since our changing, complex civilization entered the twenty-first century, the need for a harmonious approach to living is emerging as an absolute necessity. We must view the world from the top of the mountain rather than from deep in the valley. "Think Globally, Act Locally," as they say. We can all make a difference on this planet by how we choose to live our lives. As Carl Jung wrote, "It all depends on how we look at things, and not on how they are in themselves."

We must dwell on the harmony that underlies the Universe. With clarity and inner guidance, we can begin to see correlations between events and circumstances; we can see that everything works by the law of cause and effect. To expect otherwise is to have a fractured perspective and mental confusion. As my grandmother Fritzie would always remind me, "The Spirit of all life seeks expression through those individuals who, through divine love, open their hearts to one another and reflect the Light so all may live together in peace."

I am moved by the words of Chief Seattle, his warning to humanity as he surrendered his tribal lands to the U.S. Government in 1856:

> *This we know: All things are connected*
> *Like the blood which unites one family.*
> *All things are connected.*
> *Whatever befalls the Earth*
> *Befalls the sons of the Earth.*
> *Man did not weave the web of life.*
> *He is merely a strand in it.*
> *Whatever he does to the web,*
> *He does to himself.*

For peace to exist, you must first love yourself and then love each other. By simply taking loving care of ourselves, we can enrich the quality of life on this planet. *You* make a difference.

Our bodies are made up of trillions of cells; all of these cells constitute our beings. In order to maintain perfect health, each of these cells must operate at peak performance. If we have sick or weak cells, then our healthy cells must work harder so that the body as a whole can be healthy. Our planet is like a body, and we are all its individual cells. We are not separate from our fellow humans. There is no room for negative thinking, withholding forgiveness, bitterness toward others, or selfishness. What happens in one area ultimately affects the whole of the world. It is our responsibility to this body that we call our planet to be a healthy, happy, peaceful cell that radiates only goodness, positivity, oneness, and love.

Although the physical body and the body of humanity work along the same principles of harmony and cooperation, there is one difference. The cells of the body don't choose how they function. Their inherent working and functioning comes from an inner wisdom. But people do choose how they live and cooperate with one another. Harmony is not thrust upon us. We have a choice. And when we choose not to work together harmoniously, when we elect to stay separate and uncooperative, we experience collective illness—just as the body experiences disease when its components don't work well together. When we do work well together in cooperation, with compassion and peaceful hearts, we experience collective well-being—life as it is meant to be. This is the key to creating a world of peace: harmonious cooperation.

Albert Einstein is considered one of the most brilliant minds of this century. Not only was he a scientist, he was a deep-thinking metaphysician who recognized the unity and oneness behind all life. He conveys that thought in this passage:

> A human being is a part of the whole called by us
> "Universe," a part limited in time and space. He
> experiences himself, his thoughts and feelings, as
> something separated from the rest, a kind of optical
> delusion of his consciousness. This delusion is a kind
> of prison for us, restricting us to our personal desire
> and to affection for a few persons nearest to us. Our
> task must be to free ourselves from this prison by
> widening our circle of compassion to embrace all
> living creatures and the whole of nature in its beauty.

The separation and division that have so long colored our lives on this planet must be examined and corrected. To create peace on Earth, we must stop dividing the world, the nations, the races, the religions, the sexes, the ages, and the resources, and know that it's time to come together and live in harmony and love. It was Jesus who said, "Love one another" (John 13:34–35).

In his book *The Hundredth Monkey*, Ken Keyes Jr. tells of a phenomenon that scientists observed when they studied the eating habits of macaque monkeys. One monkey discovered that by washing sweet potatoes before eating them, they tasted better. She taught her mother and friends until one day there were ninety-nine monkeys who knew how to wash their sweet potatoes. The next day, when the hundredth monkey learned how to wash sweet potatoes, an amazing thing happened. The rest of the colony miraculously knew how to wash sweet potatoes, too. Not only that, but monkeys on other islands all started washing their potatoes. Keyes applies this "hundredth monkey" phenomenon to humanity. When more of us individually choose to make a difference with our lives, when we realize we do make a difference and start *acting* with that knowledge, more and more of us will hop on the bandwagon, until we reach the "millionth person" and peace spreads across the globe!

Let's take a closer look at the incredible wholeness and oneness of our bodies. On a television program not long ago, I saw something that dissolved the outer limits of my perception of wholeness and the body. It was about a study in which a woman gave a blood sample from which the white cells were isolated and then attached, with an electrode, to an electroencephalograph (EEG). The woman was then put in a room next door, not in any way connected to her extracted cells. She was asked questions, some of which evoked an emotional response. Her cells in the room next door registered the response as a weakening of the cells and a suppression of the cells' immune response. Next she was asked to go to a high-crime, dangerous area of downtown San Diego at night to see if her extracted cells could pick up her emotions from a distance of several miles. At one point, she was approached and harassed by a pimp. Immediately, her cells back in the laboratory registered her fear.

Don't ever underestimate the power of thought and the wholeness of your body, mind, and spirit. Recognize that throughout all life, there is oneness. We all share the commonality of spirit. Even scientists and theologians are now coming together to recognize and affirm the one force working behind everything.

Albert Szent-Györgyi, Nobel Prize–winning biochemist, writes about syntropy, a drive toward greater order as a fundamental principle of nature. This is an inherent drive within the life force to perfect itself and to reach higher and higher levels of organization, order, and dynamic harmony, and to move toward a synthesis of wholeness and self-perfection.

English physicist David Bohm, who was a colleague of Einstein, believed that the information of the entire universe is contained in each of its parts. Within all the separate things and events is a wholeness that is available to each part.

The way I like to approach oneness and wholeness is from a spiritual point of view. Your life is God's life. Your being and God's being are one. God is not only outside you, but within you as well. God is Omnipotent—all-powerful; God is Omniscient—knowing all things; God is Omnipresent—present in all places at the same time (He's not Omnipast!). Isn't that fantastic! It's cause for celebration.

As I said at the beginning of this chapter, we live in a busy, constantly changing, complex world. Yet beyond all the external movement, there resides a divine, unchanging, ever-present spirit that is the source of all happiness, prosperity, joy, and inner peace. We must open our hearts and receive this spirit of life. We must align ourselves with the purposes of heaven and act in accord. When we do this, we will have all the natural forces working with us, supporting us, helping us. As Ernest Holmes said:

> It is in our own heart, our own mind, our own consciousness,
> our own being, where we live twenty-four hours a day, awake or
> asleep, that that eternal share of the Infinite comes to us, because
> every man is some part of the essence of God, not as a fragment,
> but as a totality.

As a constant reminder that we are one with God and with each other, I practice the beautiful Indian salutation *Namaste*. Translated, it means, "I honor (or salute) the divinity you are (in you)." In the East, many people greet their friends and others with folded hands and the word *Namaste*. When I meet someone, I usually do this silently and without folding my hands. I inwardly acknowledge, "I honor the divinity you are." In this way, I bless myself by being reminded of the truth, and I bless others by seeing their real spiritual essence and the spiritual connection between us. This salutation sounds a note of reverence and spiritual awareness. Practiced with faith and dynamic intent, it helps to build the kind of inner attitude that manifests itself in harmonious human relations. *Namaste* is also a way to demonstrate the ability to function simultaneously at two levels—that of the personality and that of the soul. Finally, it's a gentle reminder that behind all the changes and complexities of our world, there is that omnipotent, omniscient, and *omnipresent* loving light that also resides at the center of our hearts. When you rest in that knowledge, you float in an ocean of peace.

I would like to end this chapter, and the book, with a passage from my book *The Joy Factor:*

> There can be no greater goal in life than peace. What asset could be of more value to us than unshakable calmness and tranquility? What better evidence of spiritual strength could we have than a peaceful mind and heart?
>
> Peace of mind comes from accepting what you can't control and taking responsibility for what you can. It grows out of faith in your higher power and your spiritual nature. It comes when you let go of guilt, fear, and doubt. It is the result of forgiving yourself and others for all human imperfections. When you forget the delusion that something, someday, will make you happy, you can concentrate on finding peace and contentment in the present moment. Inner peace is always in the here and now, waiting quietly for you to discover it.

Cultivate your very best life.

∿

The opposite of love is not hate, it's indifference.
The opposite of faith is not heresy, it's indifference.
The opposite of life is not death, it's indifference.

—ELIE WIESEL

Today's Affirmation & Action Step

I am lovingly connected to all beings and to all creation. I see God in everyone I meet and feel His presence in my heart and in my life. I rejoice in His oneness, knowing that I have the Spirit of life supporting me and loving me as I journey to the top of the mountain. I am one with God.

Silently greet all people today as though they are filled with radiant Light and Love. Treat them as though they are your best friends. In addition, honor and bless *you* today and respect the miraculousness of your body, your life, and the essence of who you are. Think wholeness and oneness today.

Gratitudes

Walking on Air would not have been possible without the support of Caroline Pincus, to whom this book is dedicated, and her amazing team at Conari Press. I extend my heartfelt gratitude especially to Caroline Pincus, Susie Pitzen, Lisa Trudeau, and Bonni Hamilton. Thank you also to Barb Fisher and Molly Sharp for designing the cover and interior of the book.

My deep gratitude also goes to Elline Lipkin, whose editing expertise gave my words more pizzazz and punch. She inspires me to be a better writer and is always such a joy to work with.

My appreciation is also extended to Edwin Basye, my Technical Creative Director (TCD), who moves me out of my comfort zone so I'm able to reach millions of people through my website.

To my special support system, my dear friends Ginny Swabek, Betty Wetzel, Junia Chambers, Bonnie Ross, and D & C, I thank you for your gentle and loving advice, for being my voices of reason when I needed it, and for always being there for me. (Ginny, your superb proofreading is so appreciated, too.)

To my two sisters, Jamie and June, my earth angels, whose loving support and kindness always warms my heart, lifts my spirit, and brightens my life.

Thank you to my international management team for helping orchestrate all of my projects, enterprises, and visions in North America and around the globe. Without you by my side, I would be lost. Thank you dear Faith, Emerson, Sage, Autumn, Summer, Serena, Golden, and Angela.

Finally, thank you to all of you who have supported my books and work over the years. Thanks for visiting my website frequently and for letting me know that my work inspires, uplifts, motivates, and empowers you. I am immensely grateful. Thank you so much for your positive comments and encouraging words.

About the Author

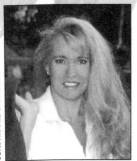

JUNIA MARIE CHAMBERS

Susan Smith Jones, PhD, has devoted her adult life to the field of holistic health and helping people unlock their potential. A health educator for over thirty years at UCLA, Susan is a widely renowned expert on fitness and nutrition, natural remedies, anti-aging, balanced living, and human potential. She has written over twenty-seven books and fifteen hundred magazine articles on these topics, including *The Joy Factor, Vegetable Soup & The Fruit Bowl* (coauthored with Dianne Warren), *Be Healthy~Stay Balanced, Renew Your Life,* and her three-book healthy eating and living set, *The Healing Power of NatureFoods, Health Bliss,* and *Recipes for Health Bliss.* She is also founder and president of Health Unlimited, a Los Angeles–based consulting firm dedicated to the advancement of peaceful, balanced living and health education.

Susan is much sought after as a culinary and holistic lifestyle coach, retreat and workshop leader, media presence, and corporate consultant. She is a frequent guest on radio and television talk shows in North America and worldwide, and she has consulted with Fortune 500 companies to create healthier workplaces, designed recipes for the natural foods industry, and guided discerning clients the world over to live their best lives.

When she is not crisscrossing the globe to deliver her message of vibrant health, she can be found hiking at sunrise and preparing delicious meals loaded with organic, plant-based foods at her home base in the Brentwood District of Los Angeles.

For more information on Susan and her work, please visit *www.SusanSmithJones.com.*

To Our Readers

Conari Press, an imprint of Red Wheel/Weiser, publishes books on topics ranging from spirituality, personal growth, and relationships to women's issues, parenting, and social issues. Our mission is to publish quality books that will make a difference in people's lives—how we feel about ourselves and how we relate to one another. We value integrity, compassion, and receptivity, both in the books we publish and in the way we do business.

Our readers are our most important resource, and we appreciate your input, suggestions, and ideas about what you would like to see published.

Please visit our website, *www.redwheelweiser.com*, to subscribe to our newsletters and learn about our upcoming books, exclusive offers, and free downloads.

You can also contact us at info@redwheelweiser.com

Conari Press
An imprint of Red Wheel/Weiser, LLC
665 Third Street, Suite 400
San Francisco, CA 94107